Adenovirus Epithelial Keratitis and Thygeson's Superficial Punctate Keratitis

Helena M. Tabery

Adenovirus Epithelial Keratitis and Thygeson's Superficial Punctate Keratitis

In Vivo Morphology in the Human Cornea

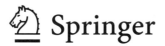 Springer

Helena M. Tabery, MD
Formerly
Ögonkliniken UMAS
20502 Malmö
Sweden
helena.tabery@telia.com

ISBN 978-3-642-21633-6   e-ISBN 978-3-642-21634-3
DOI 10.1007/978-3-642-21634-3
Springer Heidelberg Dordrecht London New York

Library of Congress Control Number: 2011937181

Printed on acid-free paper

Springer is part of Springer Science+Business Media (www.springer.com)

Preface

This book treats the in vivo morphology of human adenovirus corneal epithelial infections and of Thygeson's superficial punctate keratitis (TSPK), both captured in high-magnification photographs.

The two diseases are apparently disparate: adenovirus eye infections are very common, caused by a known agent, and highly infectious; TSPK is comparatively rare, its cause unknown, and it seems non-contagious; also, the course of the two diseases is different. Why, then, are they so often confused in clinical practice? The reason is the similarity between adenovirus epithelial infiltrates and 'coarse' TSPK epithelial lesions.

Part I of this book shows corneal epithelial changes caused by various adenovirus serotypes captured in different individuals at various points of time. The accompanying case reports highlight the importance of familiarity not only with the well-known picture of adenovirus epithelial keratitis, but also with the early manifestations of the infection. An early diagnosis is particularly difficult but of paramount importance in infections superimposed on the patients' preexisting diseases because such an event might herald a nosocomial outbreak of epidemic keratoconjunctivitis with its well-known disastrous consequences. A sequela of adenovirus epithelial keratitis are sub-epithelial opacities (infiltrates), which may persist for many years or even indefinitely; the included series shows a sequence of events occurring in them during 3 years following the infection.

Part II of this book shows corneal epithelial changes occurring in TSPK, both typical and atypical; the case reports demonstrate the long-term nature of the disease and highlight the importance of the patient's history in differentiating TSPK from adenovirus infections and, particularly so in atypical TSPK, also from herpes simplex virus infection.

The interpretation of the findings partly relates to corneal epithelial disturbances caused in human by the two other major viruses (herpes simplex and varicella-zoster) observed in vivo by the same method. Additionally, a scrutiny of sequences of events sheds some light on the mechanisms behind the similarity between epithelial changes occurring in adenovirus infections and TSPK.

I hope that this book showing the natural course of adenovirus epithelial keratitis and TSPK will not only serve as a diagnostic tool but, as no curative treatment has been found yet for either of them, also as a reference when effects of new drugs are evaluated.

Contents

About This Book

The photographs presented in this book have been chosen to show:

Part I: Adenovirus (Ad) Epithelial Keratitis

- The *in vivo morphology* of epithelial keratitis caused by various Ad serotypes, accompanying signs and sequelae (Chap. 1)
- The *in vivo morphology and dynamics* of epithelial keratitis caused by *Ad type 8* (Chap. 2)
- The *in vivo morphology and dynamics* of epithelial keratitis caused by *some other Ad serotypes* (Chap. 3)
- The *in vivo morphology and dynamics* of *subepithelial opacities/infiltrates* (Chap. 4)

Part II: Thygeson's Superficial Punctate Keratitis (TSPK)

- The *in vivo morphology* of TSPK (Chap. 5)
- The *in vivo morphology and dynamics* of *typical* TSPK (Chap. 6)
- The *in vivo morphology and dynamics* of *atypical* TSPK (Chap. 7)

The photographs were taken by *non-contact in vivo photomicrography*, a method that requires neither contact with the epithelium nor the use of anaesthetics. By this method are visualized structures that optically differ from their regularly organized surroundings; a normal corneal epithelium or stromal cells cannot be discerned. As there is no contact with the ocular surface, the architecture of epithelial changes is not disturbed by the examination, and there is no risk of spreading infections. The technique allows the use of various illumination modes to complement each other and a free application of *diagnostic dyes* to expand the information, e.g., 1% fluorescein sodium and 1% rose bengal (preservative-free solutions). These dyes are commonly used in clinical practice.

The *adenovirus diagnosis* (except for one case) was verified in conjunctival swabs by virus isolation in cell culture, and the isolates were typed by conventional neutralisation tests.

The photographs of *cell cultures* were taken by the same method.

The *bars* indicate *200 μm throughout the book.*

Abbreviations

Ad	Adenovirus
Ad	3,4,7,8 Adenovirus type
CPE	Cytopathic effect
EKC	Epidemic keratoconjunctivitis
Fluorescein	Fluorescein sodium
HSV	Herpes simplex virus
KCS	Keratoconjunctivitis sicca
TSPK	Thygeson's superficial punctate keratitis
VZV	Varicella-zoster virus

Part I

Adenovirus Epithelial Keratitis

About Adenovirus Ocular Surface Infections

Of the many *adenovirus serotypes* (at present more than 50) some cause human disease mainly involving the eye and the respiratory, gastrointestinal, and urinary tracts. Adenovirus eye infections, occurring either per se or in combination with general symptoms, are very common. The eye symptoms vary widely, ranging between a mild conjunctivitis and a severe keratoconjunctivitis leaving conjunctival scarring and disabling corneal opacities which persist for months, years, and even indefinitely. There is no curative treatment available.

The *eye symptoms* start with irritation, foreign body sensation, photophobia, and tearing in one eye; usually, within a few days, also the fellow eye becomes affected but less severely. Depending on the time elapsed between symptom onset and presentation, the eye *findings* may thus be uni- or bilateral and consist of some or all features such as: preauricular adenopathy; lid swelling with or without erythema; watery and mucoid discharge; conjunctival follicular hyperplasia, injection, chemosis, pseudomembranes, and haemorrhages; epithelial keratitis; folds of the Descemet's membrane; and anterior uveitis.

The diagnosis might be easy but also extremely difficult and there are many fallacies, for example follicular conjunctivitis clinically indistinguishable from primary herpes simplex virus infections; severe lid swelling and erythema mimicking orbital cellulitis; allergic reactions; chlamydia infections; and idiopathic anterior uveitis.

Clinically, the various serotypes cannot be distinguished from each other although a follicular conjunctivitis in combination with general symptoms such as fever and sore throat (*pharyngoconjunctival fever*) may be suspected to be caused by types 3, 4, or 7. A missed diagnosis may have serious consequences – a nosocomial transmission of *epidemic keratoconjunctivitis (EKC)*. EKC may be caused by several serotypes, but the classic cause of nosocomial infections is adenovirus type 8 (Ad8); types 19 and 37 are less common. In EKC, it is the initial stage of the infection that is particularly dangerous, not only because it is highly contagious but also because often the infection is not suspected. And a special problem, before an outbreak is discovered, are patients in whom the infection is superimposed on their preexisting diseases (Chap. 2).

The first *nosocomial outbreak of Ad8 EKC* I had the doubtful pleasure to witness occurred when I was working in the Emergency Department of the Eye Clinic. One morning, pondering over a patient with a severe keratoconjunctivitis I just had seen, I went to ask my colleagues about similar cases and the first one I met gave me an affirmative answer: Also he had just seen one. Our suspicion, sadly enough, did not result in false alarm – a large outbreak was already a fact; the ward section had to be closed down, operations stopped, and the outpatient clinics reduced to a minimum.

Some 15 years later, the outbreak happily forgotten, a similar event occurred. The suspicion arose while seeing a patient who had visited the Clinic a couple days before and now presented with a keratoconjunctivitis. At the same time, a younger colleague came to ask me to see a patient with a peculiar anterior uveitis – and the situation was clear. It was too late to avoid an outbreak, but this time it was stopped by simple precautions. Altogether, there were 33 diagnosed cases of which 23 by nosocomial transmission, mainly via fingers and a multidose bottle of eye drops used for tonometry. The outbreak was caused by Ad8.

The next occasion was a year later, but with the last outbreak fresh in mind there was only one secondary case. Also that time, the cause was Ad8.

In countries like Sweden, in which Ad8 is not endemic, the danger of an imported infection is often underestimated. Some years after the last occasion, I felt rather uncomfortable when I saw that my next patient was a Japanese gentleman who had left home with a red eye, visited the Clinic the evening before because of worsening of symptoms, and was examined by a junior staff member who failed to suspect the infection. The cause was, again, Ad8. I would like to believe that preventive measures were still working, but it might have been pure luck that at that occasion the Clinic escaped a new outbreak of EKC.

The Morphology of Adenovirus Epithelial Keratitis

Before the introduction of newer methods, the gold standard of virus detection and identification were *cell cultures* in which viruses such as adenovirus, herpes simplex (HSV), and varicella-zoster (VZV) virus cause cell swelling, bursting, and disappearance (a phenomenon termed the *virus cytopathic effect*, CPE). In *human* corneal epithelial infections, the CPE, and its impact on the epithelial architecture are clearly discernible in HSV and VZV but not so in adenovirus infections. The majority of the morphological examples shown in this chapter are of Ad8 origin (Chap. 2), but since other serotypes (Ad3, 4, 7, Chap. 3) cause the same changes, they are treated as a group.

In human adenovirus epithelial keratitis, the smallest entity detectable by the present method is a *rounded, light-reflecting cell* of about 10–15 μm in diameter, clearly abnormal to the epithelium. Distributed at random, such cells are present individually, in smaller or larger groups, and in places heaped-up. They are located superficially, within the epithelium and/or in the superficial stroma; an estimation of their exact location in depth in relation to the epithelial basement membrane is not possible in two-dimensional photographs. In time perspective, they appear early (in the present patients captured within 5 days) after the onset of symptoms, their numbers diminish with time, but they are detectable even many months and even years after the acute stage had subsided.

Larger entities are rounded vesicle- or *cyst-like structures* of about 30 μm in diameter; the surface elevations caused by them (see below) imply a location below the superficial cell layer(s); they appear early after the onset of symptoms, are amply represented during the acute stage, and disappear later on. In some corneae were additionally captured epithelial cyst, a few or several.

Fluorescein sodium visualizes that accumulations of the rounded/abnormal cells, the cyst-like structures, and some cysts cause surface elevations; all appear as dark areas, or dark spots, in the green stained tear film. Fluorescein additionally reveals superficial semi-cystic spaces appearing as brilliantly green dots; they are not numerous. Corneal surface erosion in the sense of missing substance is not a feature of adenovirus keratitis, with the (rare) exception of edematous corneae in which large epithelial areas might slough off.

Against this background stand out larger entities, the well-known adenovirus *epithelial infiltrates*, a few or several. These are rounded or somewhat irregular foci of epithelial damage measuring about 150–400 μm in diameter; their whitish appearance is partly caused by accumulations of light-reflecting rounded/abnormal cells, and partly by secondary phenomena, i.e., light-reflecting cell debris and damaged superficial epithelial cells. *Fluorescein sodium* reveals focal surface disruptions appearing as accumulated brilliantly green dots (semi-cystic spaces) in the light-reflecting areas. The staining is always circumscript, and there is no diffusion into the surroundings or the underlying stroma; adjacent surface elevations, often showing rounded/abnormal cells, appear dark in the green stained tear film. *Rose bengal* staining verifies the presence of damaged surface cells/cell debris and, as a side-effect caused by its toxic property, indirectly (with the help of fluorescein) visualizes some superficial cells. In the present patients, epithelial infiltrates were captured between 6 and 22 days after the onset of symptoms.

A *sequela* of epithelial keratitis developing in some but not all patients are subepithelial opacities usually termed subepithelial infiltrates (Chaps. 2–4).

Which of these changes is an expression of the adenovirus CPE? Although the choice is rather limited, there is no clear answer. It might be the cyst-like structures, but these are also compatible with a manifestation of epithelial edema during the acute stage and thus might represent an unspecific phenomenon. The other possibility are the rounded/abnormal cells; the problem is, however, that by the present method an incipient cell swelling, damaged cells with altered cell membranes, and invading inflammatory cells would appear the same. Hence, lacking a clear indicator, I have chosen to use purely *descriptive terms* throughout the book irrespective of their possible nature: cyst-like structures and rounded/abnormal cells.

H.M. Tabery, *Adenovirus Epithelial Keratitis and Thygeson's Superficial Punctate Keratitis*,
DOI 10.1007/978-3-642-21634-3_1, © Springer-Verlag Berlin Heidelberg 2012

Adenovirus Cytopathic Effect in Cell Cultures

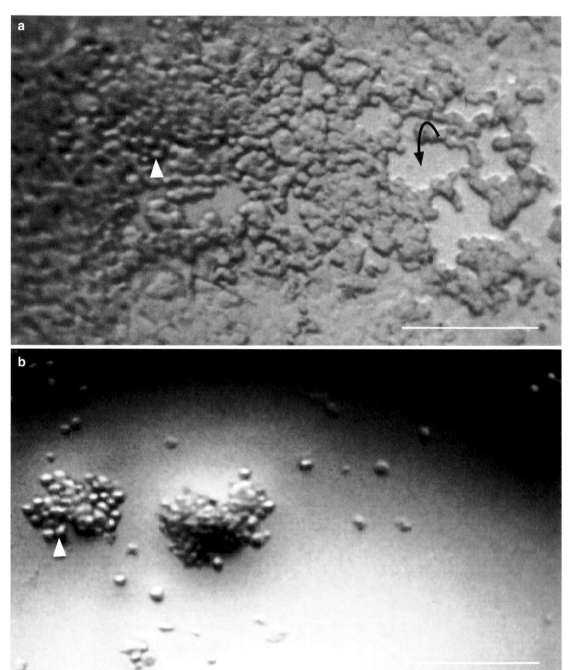

Fig. 1.1 (a, b) Cell cultures showing CPE caused by Ad8: (a) cell swelling and rounding (*arrowhead*) and cell-devoid areas (*arrow*) caused by cell disappearance, and (b) clumping of rounded/swollen cells (*arrowhead*). (Ad 589, human lung cell carcinoma)

Comment

The adenovirus in vitro CPE does not have any clearly discernible in vivo counterpart; in vivo, a loss of substance does not occur, and the nature of the rounded/abnormal cells (cf. Fig. 1.2, opposite page) is unclear.

Rounded/Abnormal Cells in Human Adenovirus Epithelial Keratitis

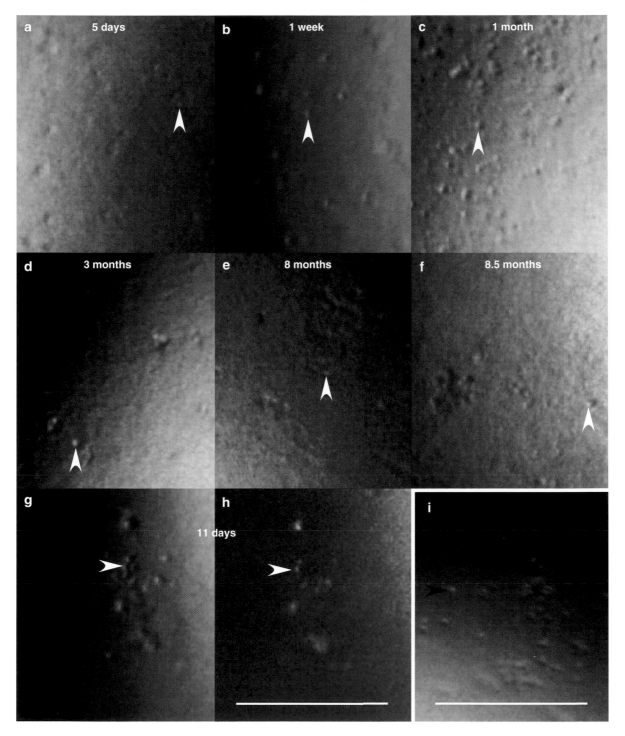

Fig. 1.2 (a–h) Rounded/abnormal cells (*arrowheads*), individual or grouped, captured in different individuals at various points of time after symptom onset: (a) 5 days, Ad8; (b) 1 week, Ad4; (c) 1 month, Ad8; (d) 3 months, Ad8; (e) 8 months, Ad8; (f) 8.5 months, Ad8; (g, h) 11 days, Ad8; (h) shows the light-reflecting property of the rounded/abnormal cells (the *arrowheads* in g and h are placed in corresponding locations). For further examples see Chap. 2–4. (i) For comparison, inflammatory cells (*arrowhead*) on the endothelium in anterior uveitis unrelated to adenovirus infection

Cyst-Like Structures; Fluorescein Staining

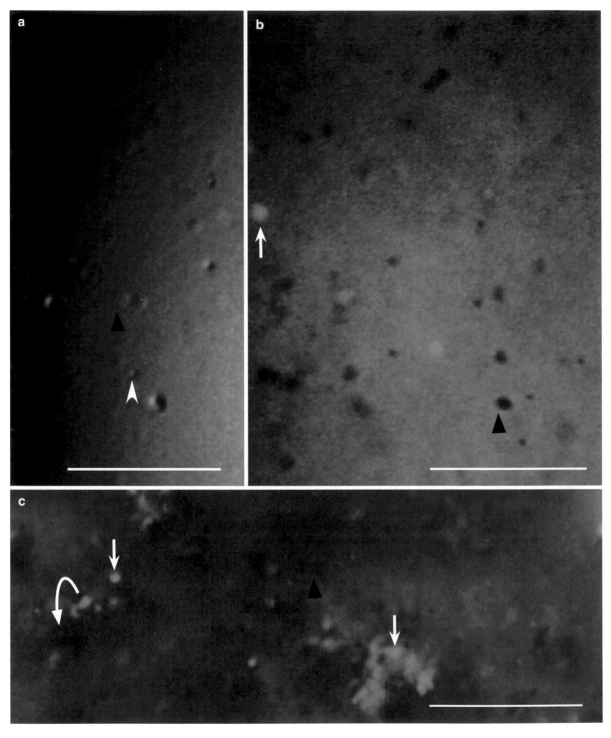

Fig. 1.3 (a) Cyst-like structures (*black arrowhead*) and rounded/abnormal cells (*white arrowhead*) 1 week after symptom onset (Ad4). (b) Protruding cyst-like structures (*arrowhead*) appear dark in the green stained tear film. The brilliantly green dot (*arrow*) indicates fluorescein penetration into a semi-cystic space (5 days after symptom onset; Ad8). (c) Brilliantly green dots (*straight arrows*), individual or grouped, and smaller (*arrowhead*) or larger (*bowed arrow*) surface elevations appearing dark in the green stained tear film (17 days after symptom onset; Ad8)

Fluorescein and Rose Bengal Staining

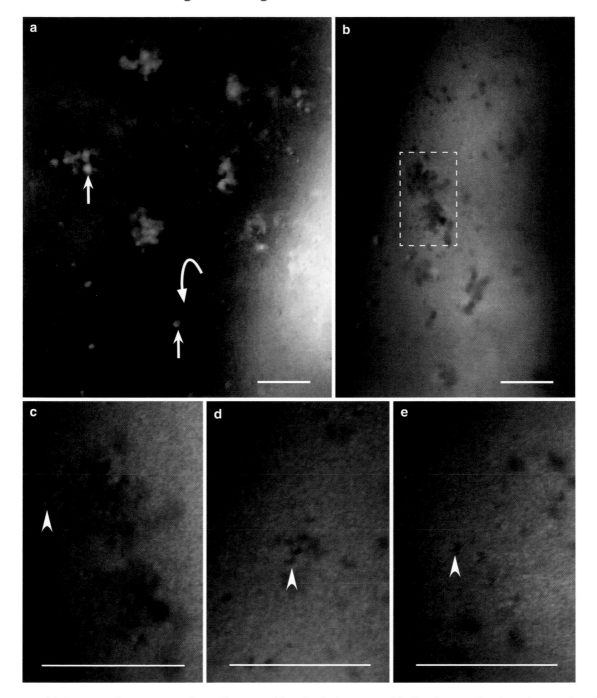

Fig. 1.4 (a) Survey. In the green stained tear film are visible individual or grouped brilliantly green dots (*straight arrows*) and surface elevations (dark; *bowed arrow*) (17 days after symptom onset; Ad8). (b) Survey. Rose bengal stains damaged surface cells/cell debris red. The area *in frame* is shown at higher magnification in (c). (c–e) Only damaged superficial cells stain red; the rounded/abnormal cells (*arrowheads*) do not stain. (11 days after symptom onset; Ad8)

Comment

In this patient, some rose bengal staining in the in-between areas was possibly relatable to a (probably preexisting) dry eye; because of its stinging property, the dye was used only in a few patients.

Epithelial Infiltrates 1

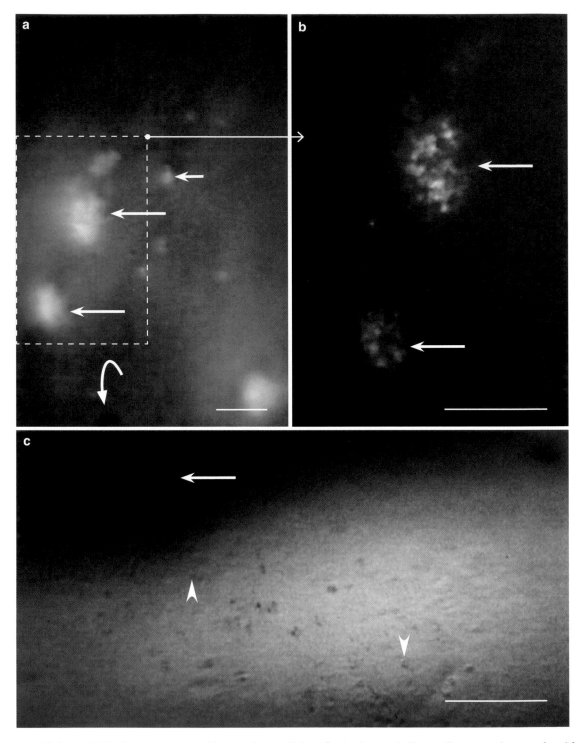

Fig. 1.5 (a) Survey. With fluorescein are visible several larger light-reflecting lesions/infiltrates (*long arrows*), green dots (*short arrow*), and surface elevations (*bowed arrow*). The area in *frame* is shown at higher magnification in b. (b) The infiltrates (*arrows*) show green fluorescein stained dots visible between damaged surface cells/cell debris staining red with rose bengal; there is no fluorescein diffusion into the surroundings. (The long arrows in a and b are placed in corresponding locations.) (c) Many rounded/abnormal cells (*arrowheads*) are present in the in-between areas; the *arrow* points to an additional infiltrate. (12 days after symptom onset; Ad8)

Epithelial Infiltrates 2

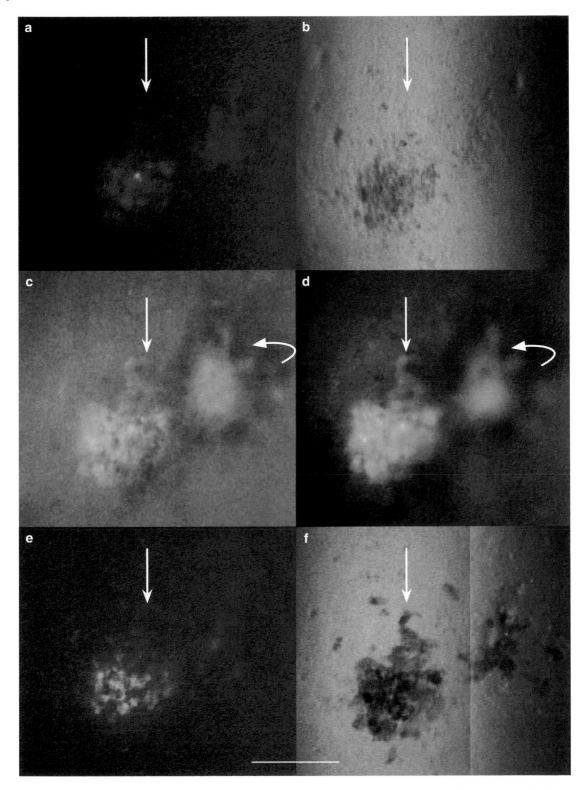

Fig. 1.6 (a–f) Various aspects of epithelial infiltrates (*arrows*): (a) light-reflecting property, (b) granular appearance, (c, d) circum-script fluorescein staining and surface elevations (*dark*, *bowed arrows*), (e) absence of fluorescein diffusion, and (e, f) rose bengal staining of damaged surface cells/cell debris ((f) is a composed photograph). (12 days after symptom onset; Ad8. The markers are placed in corresponding locations)

Addendum 1. Toxic Effect of Rose Bengal Dye

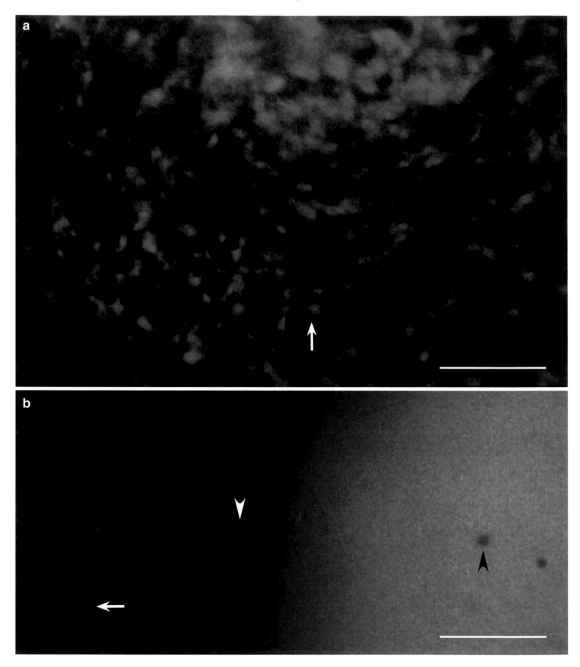

Fig. 1.7 (**a**) In this cornea, before staining, the surface epithelium seemed normal and with fluorescein showed only a few green dots; after the application of rose bengal myriads of variously shaped green dots appeared (*arrow*). (**b**) shows a different area of the same cornea; to the left is visible green fluorescein staining (*arrow*), to the right a minimal rose bengal staining (*black arrowhead*), and in the center a group of rounded/abnormal cells (*white arrowhead*). (6 weeks after symptom onset; Ad8)

Comment

This phenomenon is a manifestation of the toxic effect of rose bengal. The dye seems to cause disruptions of intercellular junctions, and the (transparent) superficial cells are indirectly visualized by penetration of green stained tear fluid below them.

Addendum 2. Conjunctival Changes

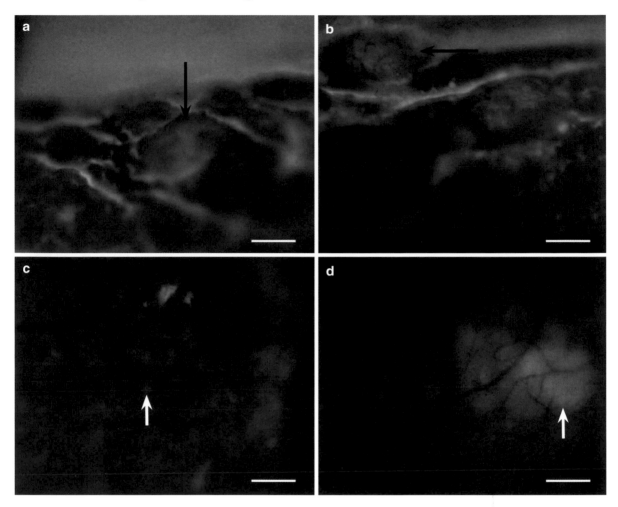

Fig. 1.8 (**a, b**) Follicles (*arrows*) in the lower fornix, (**c**) punctate fluorescein staining (*arrow*), and (**d**) larger fluorescein stained spots on the conjunctiva, all occurring in adenovirus ocular surface infections; these changes are unspecific. (Fluorescein sodium, blue filter)

Fig. 1.9 (*Right*) Subepithelial opacities/infiltrates 2 months after symptom onset (Ad4). This phenomenon is treated in Chaps. 2–4

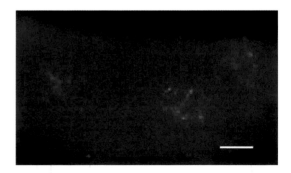

Adenovirus Type 8 Epithelial Keratitis: The Development, Accompanying Signs, and Sequelae

2

This chapter shows the development of Ad8 keratitis in patients of whom all but one (Case 8) were exposed to the virus during a nosocomial outbreak of EKC. The infection was transmitted either directly in the Clinic or by infected contacts. Since in clinical practice infections with various adenovirus serotypes cannot be distinguished from each other, Ad8 can serve as a model of a sequence events common to all of them. In the absence of causative treatment, the cases presented in this chapter show the natural course of the disease. Cortisone eye drops were not used except for a couple of days during the acute stage in one patient (Case 8) because of an initial diagnostic error.

In *time perspective*, lacking better indicators, the duration of the keratitis at presentation is related to the onset of symptoms as reported by the patient, which of course does not tell when exactly during the course of the disease the corneal epithelium became affected. It might have occurred early, as shown in Case 1 presenting about 30 h. after the onset of symptoms.

The morphological components of adenovirus epithelial keratitis are few (Chap. 1) and the *course of the disease* rather stereotype: first to appear are superficial cyst-like structures; either concurrently with them, or shortly thereafter, appear rounded/abnormal cells, individual or grouped. During the next few days, the numbers of both tend to increase, and the rounded/abnormal cells show propensity to heap-up; this phenomenon eventually results in larger lesions termed adenovirus *epithelial infiltrates*. The cyst-like structures are first to clear. The numbers of rounded/abnormal cells, on the other hand, diminish only slowly, and in some patients they persist for many months or even years after the acute disease had subsided.

These are patients who develop a *sequela* of adenovirus epithelial keratitis termed *subepithelial infiltrates*. Clinically, this denomination seems to apply to *light-reflecting flecks or opacities,* mild or dense, few or many, present after the integrity of the epithelial surface has been restored as judged by the absence of fluorescein staining. Published *histological preparations* have shown subepithelial accumulations of inflammatory cells, but at what point of time the subepithelial stroma becomes involved seems unknown. In vivo, there is no abrupt change, there is the same cellular component as before, and the only indicators of subepithelial involvement are structures implying damage to the lamellar composition of the superficial stroma the initial stages of which are difficult to detect. Since the cells appear the same during the course of the disease, I have chosen (Chap. 1) to use the purely descriptive term rounded/abnormal cells irrespective of their possible nature throughout the book. Concerning the subepithelial infiltrates, the *terminology* is even more challenging. After having pondered the question for a while, I found it practical to use the term in accordance with the clinical application, i.e., also in cases in which no clear subepithelial stromal involvement has been captured. The substructure, the superficial location, and the development of subepithelial infiltrates are shown in Case 10 (cf. also Chap. 4).

Diagnostic errors occurring during the period of time elapsing between symptom onset and (in the context) the diagnostic adenovirus epithelial infiltrates highlight the importance of familiarity with the appearance of the early corneal manifestations: With the slit lamp, the cornea appears dusty but not lustreless; a careful observation discloses the presence of light-reflecting dots and, with fluorescein sodium, many surface elevations. If attention is not paid, patients with *accompanying signs* of anterior uveitis are easily diagnosed with primary uveitis, particularly those with a history of a recurrent one (Cases 3 and 8). Very tricky are also nosocomial infections superimposed on preexisting corneal epithelial diseases (Cases 9 and 10); before an outbreak is discovered, they tend to be erroneously attributed to allergic reactions to treatment.

H.M. Tabery, *Adenovirus Epithelial Keratitis and Thygeson's Superficial Punctate Keratitis,* DOI 10.1007/978-3-642-21634-3_2, © Springer-Verlag Berlin Heidelberg 2012

Case 1: EKC: An Occupational Hazard

Case Report

A 40-year-old woman presented with irritation, foreign body sensation, tearing, and redness of the right eye, all starting about 30 h. before examination. The lids were slightly swollen, the eye moderately injected, the conjunctiva showed follicular hyperplasia and, with fluorescein sodium, myriads of green dots; with the slit lamp, the corneal epithelium appeared slightly hazy. The left eye was white. Adenovirus infection was suspected. The fellow eye became affected 3 days later but less severely.

The photographs of the right cornea were taken at presentation and 5, 12, and 20 days, and 2 months after the onset of symptoms.

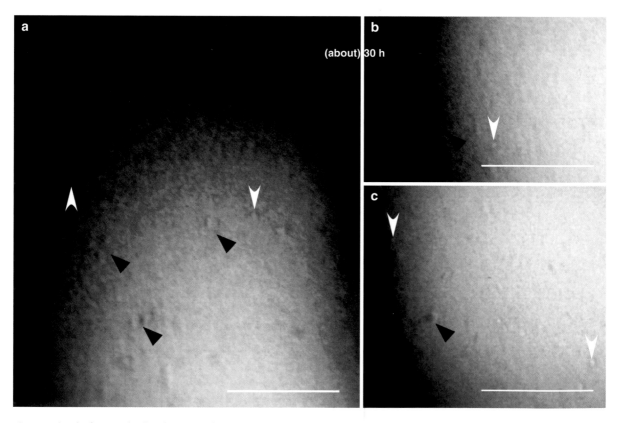

Fig. 2.1   (a–c) About 30 h after the onset of symptoms, the corneal epithelium shows discrete rounded cyst-like structures (*black arrowheads*). The smaller structures (*white arrowheads*) might represent rounded/abnormal cells (cf. Fig. 2.2, *opposite page*)

Comment

It is uncommon to see a patient presenting that early after the onset of symptoms. This patient was a staff member whose symptoms had started during a just discovered outbreak of nosocomial infection.

EKC: An Occupational Hazard (Case 1, cont.)

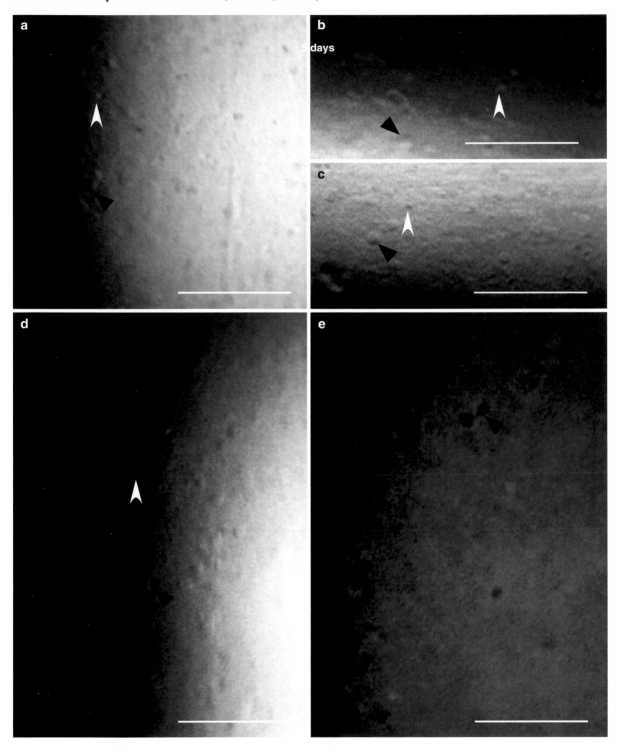

Fig. 2.2 (a–e) Five days after symptom onset. In (a–d) are visible rounded/abnormal cells (*white arrowheads*) and many rounded cyst-like structures (*black arrowheads*) which (e) are protruding (dark; *arrowheads*) in the tear film stained green with fluorescein. (Cf. Figs. 2.6 and 2.7)

EKC: An Occupational Hazard (Case 1, cont.)

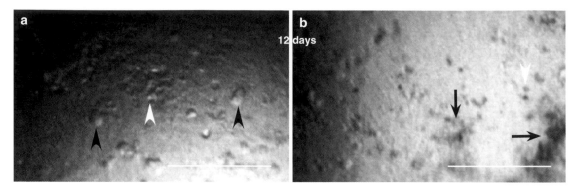

Fig. 2.3 (**a**, **b**) Twelve days after symptom onset, the epithelium is heavily disturbed. It shows many rounded/abnormal cells (*white arrowheads*), individual or grouped, and distinct epithelial cysts (*black arrowheads*). In places, the cells seem mixed with cell debris (**b**, *arrows*). (Adapted from [4])

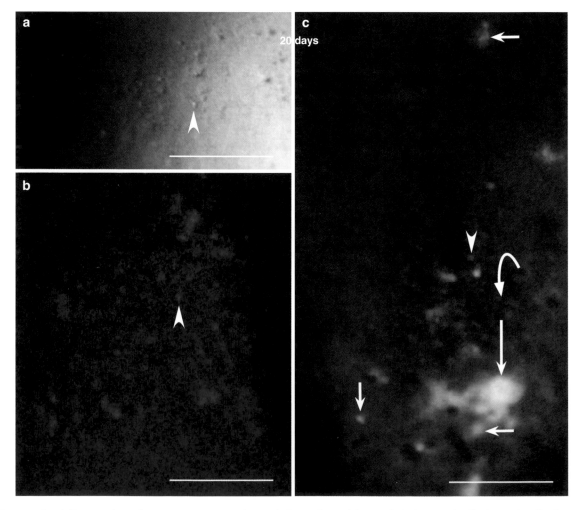

Fig. 2.4 (**a–c**) Twenty days after symptom onset, the epithelium shows (**a**) rounded/abnormal cells (*arrowhead*); they are (**b**, **c**) light reflecting (*arrowheads*). (**c**) With fluorescein are visible brilliantly green dots, individual (*short arrows*) or grouped (*long arrow*), and surface elevations (dark; *bowed arrow*)

EKC: An Occupational Hazard (Case 1, cont.)

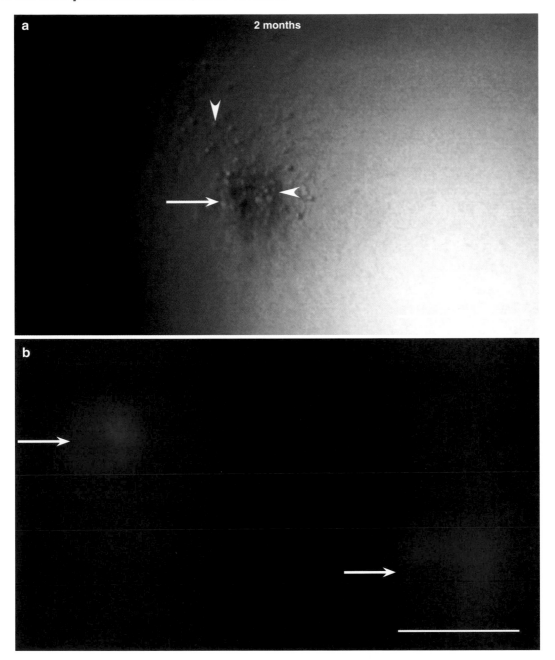

Fig. 2.5 (**a, b**) Two months after symptom onset (**a**) a lesion (*arrow*) that contains rounded/abnormal cells (*arrowhead*) is visible; such cells (*arrowhead*) are also present outside it. (**b**) Two lesions staining green with fluorescein (blue filter)

Comment

Sometimes, new surface disruptions occur long after the surface has been restored. Cf. Figs. 4.14 and 4.27.

Addendum

This patient developed dense subepithelial opacities/infiltrates that only gradually faded away.

Case 2: A Sequel of a Friendly Visit

Case Report

A 77-year-old man was referred to the Eye Clinic by a general practitioner because of a left-sided conjunctivitis of 4 days duration. The left eye was injected, the conjunctiva swollen, and the cornea showed many dust-like epithelial dots and folds of the Descemet's membrane. The right eye was white. Adenovirus was suspected. The following day, the patient presented again because of worsening of symptoms. The right eye was slightly injected and showed many follicles in the lower fornix, and the symptoms in the left eye were more severe. The source of the infection was traced to a contact with a close friend who had contracted nosocomial infection.

Three months after onset, the right cornea showed two discrete subepithelial opacities/infiltrates and the left cornea several dense ones. 7.5 months after onset, the right cornea was clear and the periphery of left one showed a few discrete subepithelial opacities.

The photographs of the left cornea were taken 5 and 19 days, and 3 and 7.5 months after the onset of symptoms.

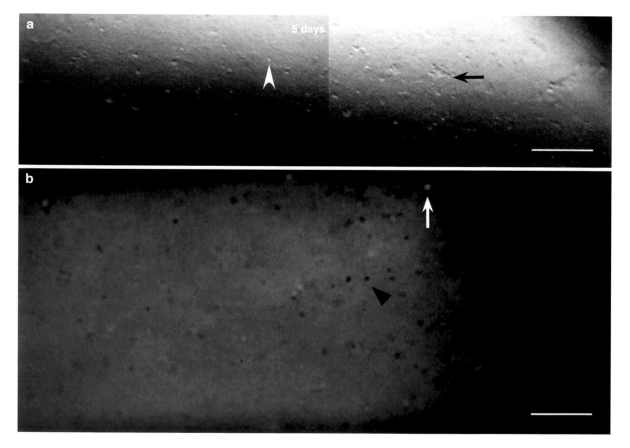

Fig. 2.6 (a, b) Five days after symptom onset. Survey. (a) Without staining, the epithelium shows many fine dots spread over the surface, individual (*arrowhead*) or grouped (*arrow*). (Composed photograph.) (b) With fluorescein are visible many rounded dark (*arrowhead*) and some brilliantly green (*arrow*) dots. For details see Fig. 2.7 (*opposite page*)

A Sequel of a Friendly Visit (Case 2, cont.)

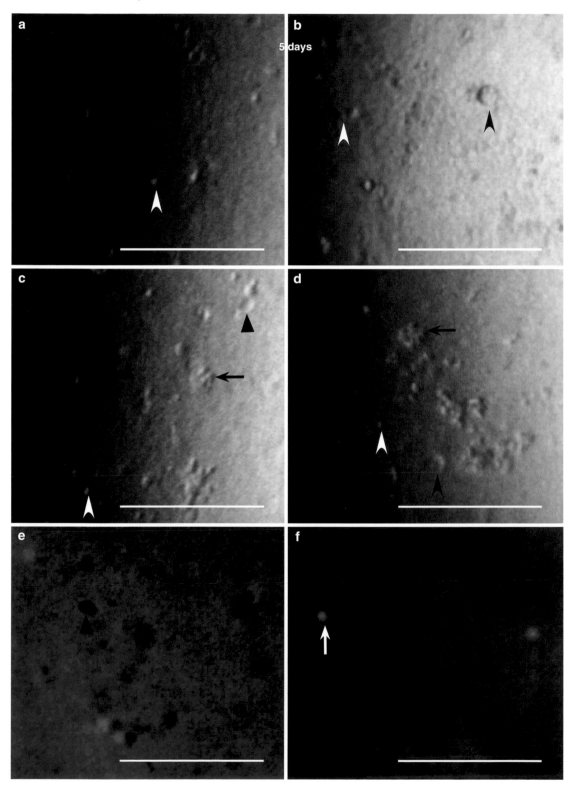

Fig. 2.7 (**a–f**) The cornea shown in Fig. 2.6. Visible are (**a–d**) rounded/abnormal cells, individual (*white arrowheads*) or grouped (*arrows*), (**c**) cyst-like changes (*black arrowheads*), and (**b** and **d**) epithelial cysts (*black arrowheads*). (**e, f**) With fluorescein are visible small protrusions (dark; *arrowheads*) in the green stained tear film and a few green dots (*arrow*)

A Sequel of a Friendly Visit (Case 2, cont.)

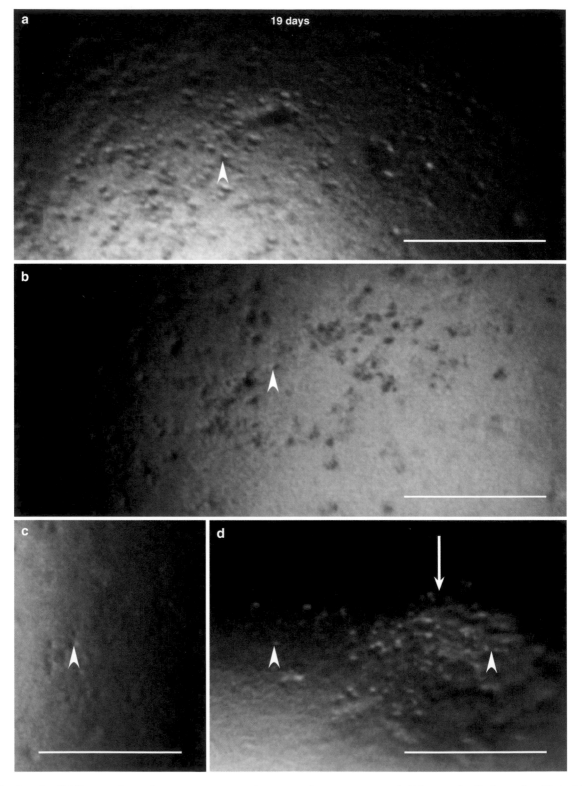

Fig. 2.8 (a–d) Nineteen days after symptom onset, the cornea shows many rounded/abnormal cells (*arrowheads*), in (d) heaped-up in a distinct epithelial infiltrate (*arrow*). (d adapted from [4])

A Sequel of a Friendly Visit (Case 2, cont.)

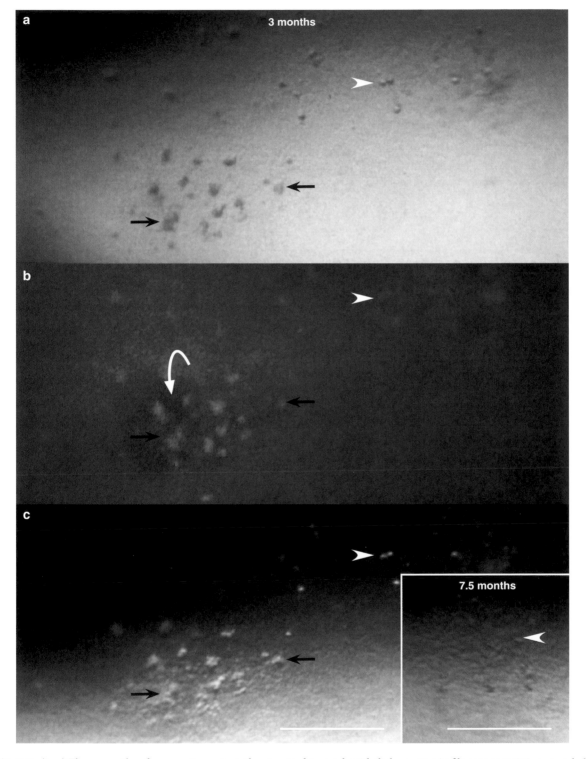

Fig. 2.9 (a–c) Three months after symptom onset, the cornea shows subepithelial opacities/infiltrates containing rounded/abnormal cells, individual (*arrowheads*) or grouped (*black arrows*); (b) shows their light-reflecting property and a surface elevation (dark; *bowed arrow*). (The black arrows and the arrowheads are placed in corresponding locations.) *Inset*: rounded/abnormal cells (*arrowhead*) present 7.5 months after onset

Case 3: Anterior Uveitis and Nosocomial Infection

Case Report

A 74-year-old woman treated with cortisone eye drops for right-sided anterior uveitis. Nine days after the last visit, she presented again because of augmenting redness and irritation in the fellow eye. Both eyes were slightly injected and the corneae showed discrete dust-like epithelial dots. Four days later, when the lids were swollen and the corneae additionally showed folds of the Descemet's membrane, adenovirus was suspected. Six weeks after symptom onset, the eyes were white and the corneae clear. She never developed subepithelial opacities/infiltrates.

The photographs of the left cornea were taken 9 and 15 days after the onset of symptoms.

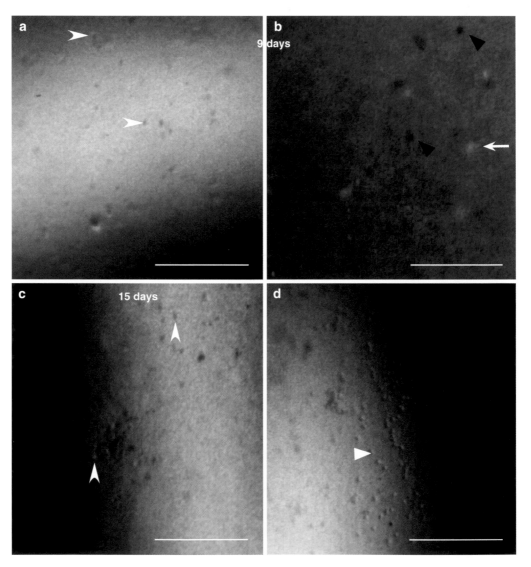

Fig. 2.10 (**a–d**) Nine days after symptom onset, the cornea shows (**a**) rounded/abnormal cells (*arrowheads*) and (**b**) rounded protrusions (dark; *arrowheads*) and green dots (*arrow*) in the tear film stained green with fluorescein. (**c**) Rounded/abnormal cells (*arrowheads*), in places grouped (*arrow*) are still present 15 days after onset. (**d**) shows, for comparison, inflammatory cells (*arrowhead*) attached to the endothelium during a mild anterior uveitis present 15 days after the onset of symptoms relatable to Ad8 infection

Case 4: A Case of a Caring Wife

Case Report

This 87-year-old woman, who had administered eye drops to her husband with nosocomial infection, presented with bilateral keratoconjunctivitis 4 days after symptom onset. She developed many subepithelial opacities/infiltrates still present 2 years later.

The photographs of the left cornea were taken 17 days after symptom onset.

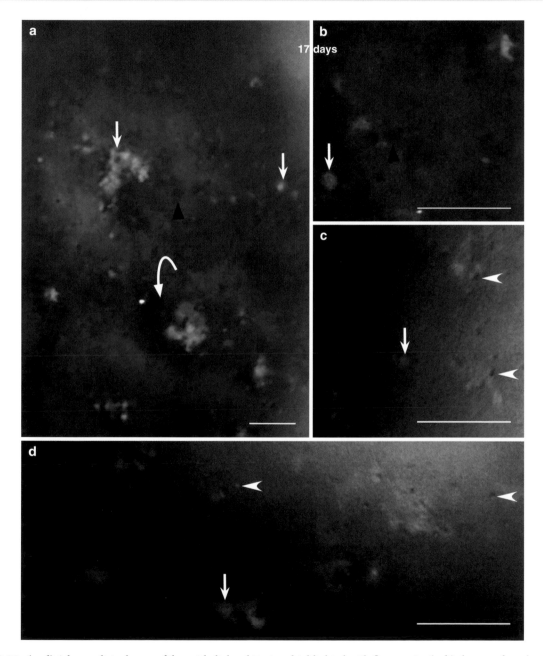

Fig. 2.11 (**a–d**) A heavy disturbance of the epithelial architecture highlighted with fluorescein. (**a, b**) show surface elevations (dark; *bowed arrow* and *arrowheads*) and brilliantly green dots (*straight arrows*). In (**c, d**) are visible green dots (*arrows*) and rounded/abnormal cells (*arrowheads*)

Case 5: Nosocomial Infection After Suture Removal

Case Report

A 85-year-old woman presented with irritation and foreign body sensation in her left eye. An old corneal suture after a previous cataract operation was removed. Sixteen days later she presented again, this time because of irritation and redness in both eyes that had started a week earlier (9 days after her first visit). The lids were swollen, the conjunctivae injected and swollen, and the corneae showed fine epithelial dots and folds of the Descemet's membrane. Nosocomial adenovirus infection was suspected. She developed discrete subepithelial opacities/infiltrates in both corneae; only a few very faint ones with no visual consequences were present 7 months after symptom onset.

The photographs of the left cornea were taken 2 weeks, 4 weeks, and 7 months after the onset of symptoms.

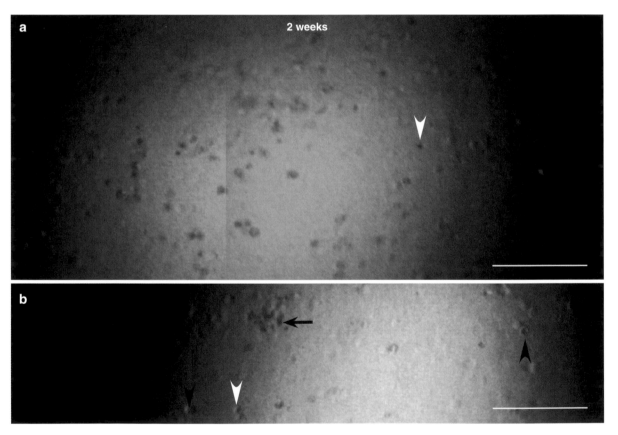

Fig. 2.12 (**a, b**) Survey of corneal epithelial changes captured 2 weeks after the onset of symptoms. The epithelium shows many rounded/abnormal cells (*white arrowheads*), in places grouped (*arrow*), and many small cysts (*black arrowheads*) spread over the surface (composed photographs). For details see Fig. 2.13 (*opposite page*)

Nosocomial Infection After Suture Removal (Case 5, cont.)

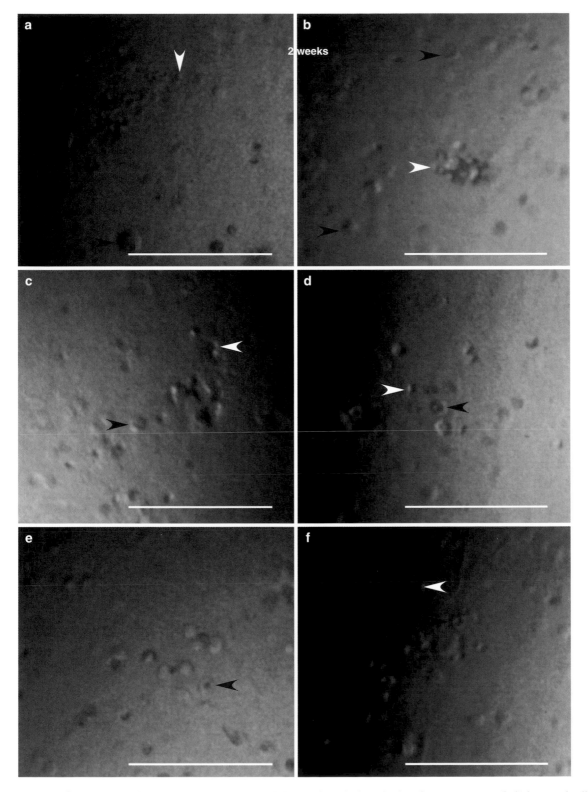

Fig. 2.13 (a–f) Two weeks after symptom onset. The epithelium is heavily disturbed. It shows many rounded/abnormal cells (*white arrowheads*) and small cysts (*black arrowheads*); of these, many contain a rounded cell. (This phenomenon is unspecific)

Nosocomial Infection After Suture Removal (Case 5, cont.)

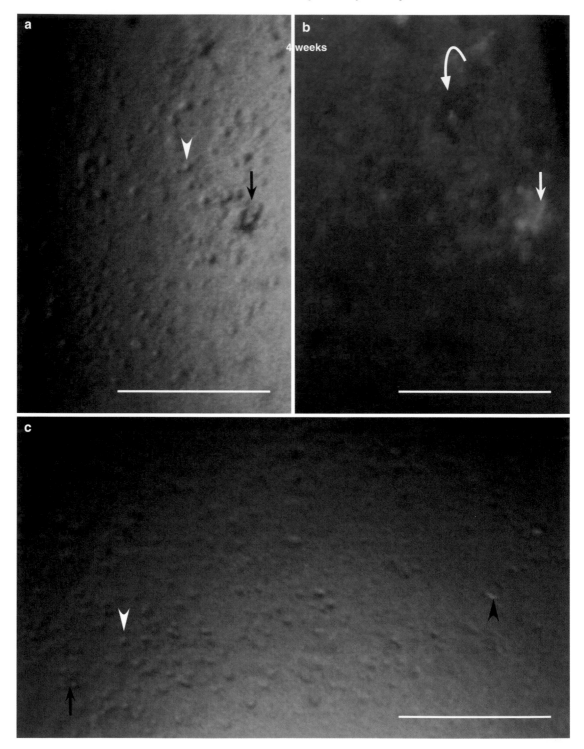

Fig. 2.14 (a–c) Four weeks after symptom onset, the epithelium shows (a and c) many rounded/abnormal cells, individual (*white arrowheads*) or grouped (*arrows*) and a cyst (*black arrowhead*). (b) In the tear film stained green with fluorescein are visible surface elevations (dark; *bowed arrow*) and brilliantly green dots (*short arrow*)

Nosocomial Infection After Suture Removal (Case 5, cont.)

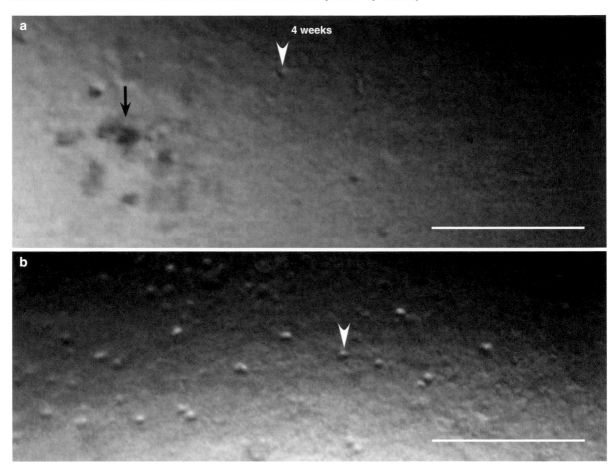

Fig. 2.15 (a, b) Different areas of the same cornea as in Fig. 2.14 showing rounded/abnormal cells (*arrowheads*); in the group indicated by *arrow*, the cells seem mixed with cell debris

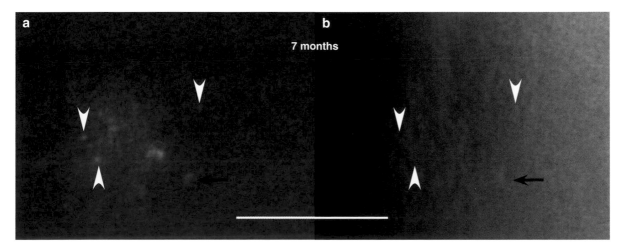

Fig. 2.16 (a, b) Seven months after epithelial keratitis the cornea shows (a) faint subepithelial opacities /infiltrates containing a few light-reflecting rounded/abnormal cells, individual (*arrowheads*) or grouped (*arrows*). (The markers are placed in corresponding locations)

Case 6: Nosocomial Infection After Applanation Tonometry

Case Report

Six days after a visit to the Eye Clinic, a 62-year-old woman with glaucoma woke up with redness and irritation in the left eye. The eye was slightly injected and the lower fornix showed follicular hyperplasia; the cornea appeared normal. A week later, both eyes were injected and within a further 5 days developed many corneal epithelial infiltrates. Sixteen months after onset, the left cornea showed many dense subepithelial opacities/infiltrates.

The photographs of the left cornea were taken 12 days and 7 weeks after the onset of symptoms.

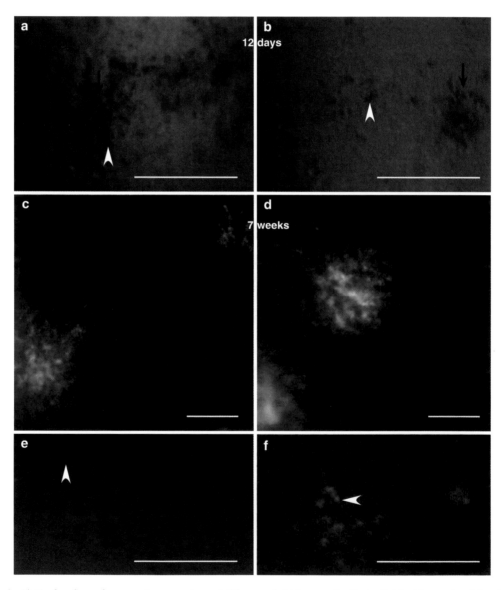

Fig. 2.17 (**a**, **b**) Twelve days after symptom onset are visible rounded/abnormal cells, individual (*arrowheads*) or heaped-up and apparently mixed with cell debris (*arrows*). (**c**, **d**) Subepithelial opacities/infiltrates 7 weeks after symptom onset (*arrows*). (**e**) Rounded/abnormal cells, individual (*arrowhead*) or grouped (*arrow*) are (**f**) light-reflecting (*arrowhead*). (Cf. Figs. 2.4, 2.21, 2.26, 2.27)

Case 7: A Woman Infected by a Caring Relative

Case Report

To this 77-year-old woman, the virus was transmitted by a relative (herself mother of a patient with noso-comial infection) who was nursing her. She suffered a severe bilateral keratoconjunctivitis starting in the left eye and subsequently developed many subepithelial opacities/infiltrates interfering with vision in both eyes.

The photographs of the left cornea were taken 4 weeks and 17 months after the onset of symptoms.

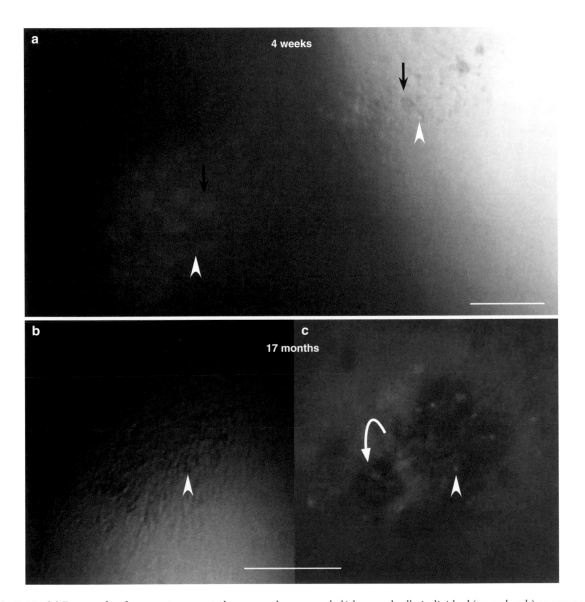

Fig. 2.18 (**a**) Four weeks after symptom onset, the cornea shows rounded/abnormal cells, individual (*arrowheads*) or grouped (*arrows*). (**b–c**) Subepithelial opacities/infiltrates containing rounded/abnormal cells (*arrowheads*) 17 months after onset. In (**c**) are visible surface elevations (*dark*, *arrow*) present in the same area as in (**b**); the surface appears intact. (The arrowheads are placed in corresponding locations)

Case 8: A Potential Source of a Nosocomial Outbreak

Case Report

In a 76-year-old woman with a history of recurrent bilateral anterior uveitis and corneal marginal infiltrations, an incipient adenovirus infection was confused with an incipient recurrence of anterior uveitis. She stopped using steroid eye drops after a few days because of symptom worsening. At presentation, 10 days later, both eyes were injected, and the corneae showed dust-like epithelial keratitis; the right cornea additionally showed folds of the Descemet's membrane. Adenovirus was suspected; laboratory tests revealed Ad8.

The photographs of the left cornea were taken 11 and 20 days after the onset of symptoms.

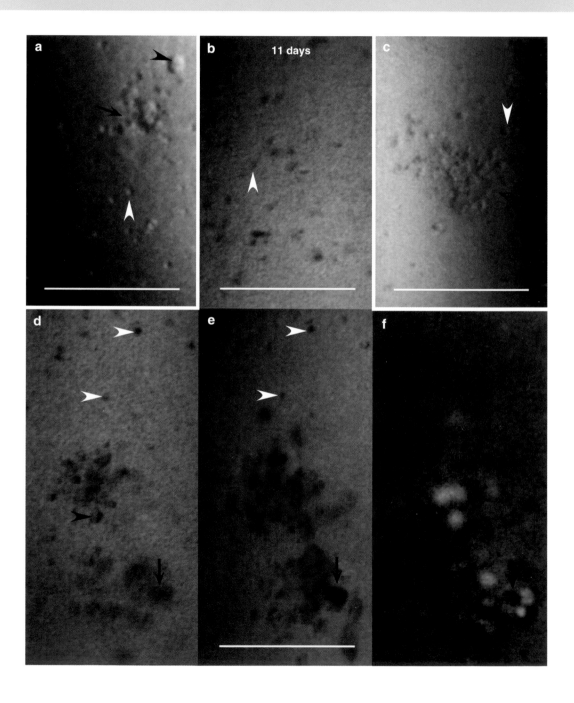

A Potential Source of a Nosocomial Outbreak (Case 8, cont.)

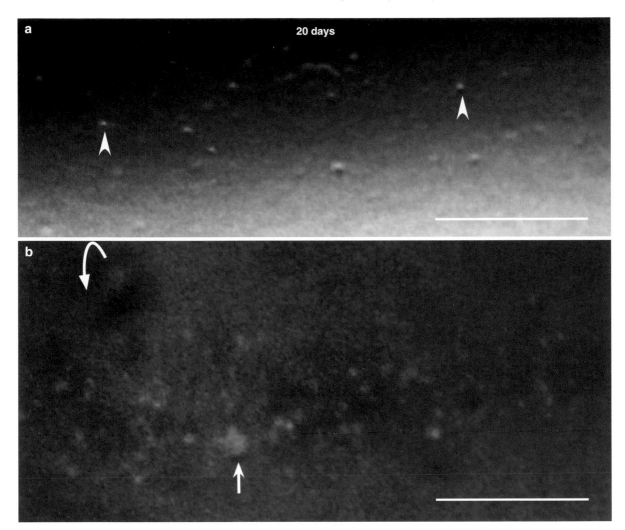

Fig. 2.20 (a, b) Twenty days after symptom onset, the cornea still shows (a) many rounded/abnormal cells (*arrowheads*) and (b), with fluorescein, surface elevations (*bowed arrow*) and a few green stained dots (*short arrow*)

Addendum

The patient had acquired the infection in Central Europe. With an outbreak of nosocomial Ad8 infection fresh in mind, the awareness of the danger was still high and there was only one secondary case.

The patient was followed for a further 1.5 years because of recurrent anterior uveitis. She developed only one very faint peripheral subepithelial opacity. Dry eye was diagnosed 4 months after the infection.

Fig. 2.19 (a–f) (*Opposite page*) Eleven days after symptom onset. The epithelium shows (a–d) many rounded/abnormal cells, individual (*white arrowheads*) or grouped (*arrows*) and a cyst (*black arrowhead*). (e, f) Show the same area as (d). (e) Damaged surface cells stain red with rose bengal. (f) Between red stained cells are visible fluorescein stained dots (green, *arrowhead*). (The markers are placed in corresponding locations)

Case 9: Nosocomial Infection in a Contact Lens Wearer

Case Report

A 28-year-old contact lens wearer presented in the Emergency Department because of irritation and redness in both eyes. At that occasion, and 4 days later, the corneal epithelium showed unspecific superficial changes suggestive of contact lens overwear. Six days after the second visit he presented again because of symptom worsening in both eyes. The corneal epithelium showed only a fine epitheliopathy but there were new findings: lid swelling, follicular hyperplasia, conjunctival injection, all severe, and a painful swelling of a preauricular lymph node. These findings were strongly suggestive of adenovirus infection. A week later, the symptoms were less severe but both corneae showed many epithelial infiltrates.

The photographs of the left cornea were taken at that occasion, about 10 days after the onset of symptoms relatable to adenovirus infection.

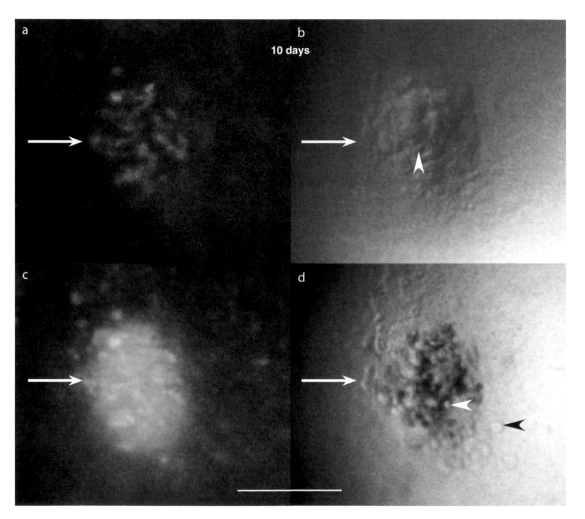

Fig. 2.21 (**a–d**) This epithelial infiltrate (*arrows*), captured about 10 days after symptom onset (**a**) is light-reflecting, (**b**) contains rounded/abnormal cells (*arrowhead*), (**c**) shows a circumscript green fluorescein staining, and (**d**) red rose bengal staining of damaged superficial cells/cell debris. In (**d**) are also visible rounded/abnormal cells (*white arrowhead*) and a few adjacent cysts or cyst-like structures (*black arrowhead*). (The arrows are placed in corresponding locations)

Nosocomial Infection in a Contact Lens Wearer (Case 9, cont.)

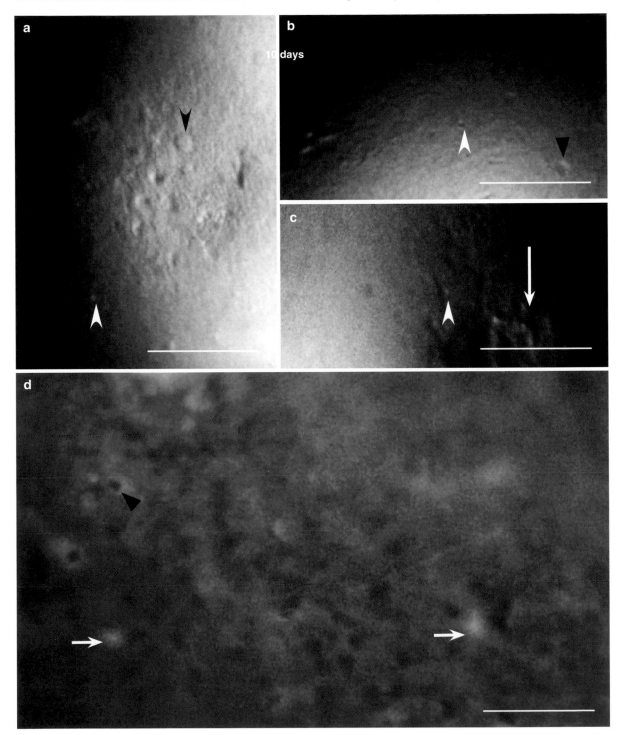

Fig. 2.22 (**a–d**) Different areas of the same cornea as in Fig. 2.21 show (**a–c**) rounded/abnormal cells (*white arrowheads*) and cysts or cyst-like structures (*black arrowheads*). In (**c**) is additionally visible a part of an epithelial infiltrate (*arrow*), and in (**d**), with fluorescein, many small surface elevations (*dark; arrowhead*) and a few brilliantly green dots (*arrows*)

Case 10: Nosocomial Infection in Corneal Erosion

Case Report

A 53-year-old woman was pecked in her left eye by her pet bird. A clean epithelial erosion was treated with antibiotic ointment. Seventeen days later, she was referred by a practitioner back to the Eye Clinic because symptom worsening. In the left eye, the lids were swollen, the conjunctiva injected and swollen, and the cornea showed a large erosion; the remaining epithelium was swollen and there were folds of the Descemet's membrane. In addition, she had symptoms also in the fellow eye, for 4 days; that eye was moderately injected and the corneal epithelium appeared dusty. Nosocomial Ad8 infection was suspected. After a further 2 days, the right cornea showed epithelial infiltrates. The erosion in the left eye healed within a further 3 days, but the cornea started to show many epithelial infiltrates. Dense subepithelial opacities/infiltrates interfering with vision developed in both corneae; they were still present a year after the infection.

The photographs of the right (not traumatized) cornea were taken 6 and 7 days; 4, 6, and 9 weeks; 3, 5, and 8 months; and 1 year after the onset of symptoms.

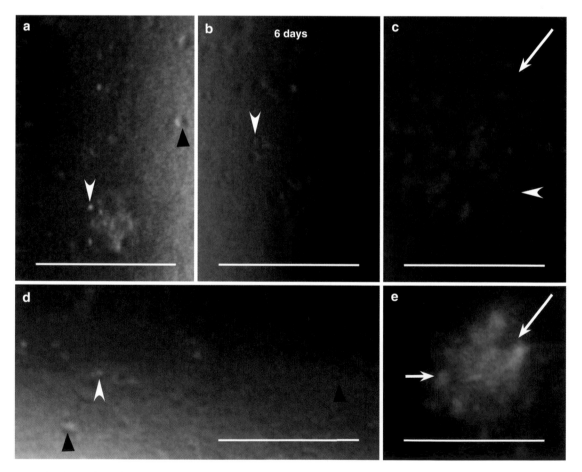

Fig. 2.23 (a–d) Six days after symptom onset, the epithelium shows many rounded/abnormal cells (*white arrowheads*), individual or heaped-up (c, *arrow*) and cyst-like structures (*black arrowheads*). (e) With fluorescein, the surface of an infiltrate (*long arrow*) shows brilliantly green dots (*short arrow*); there is no diffusion into the surroundings

Nosocomial Infection in Corneal Erosion (Case 10, cont.)

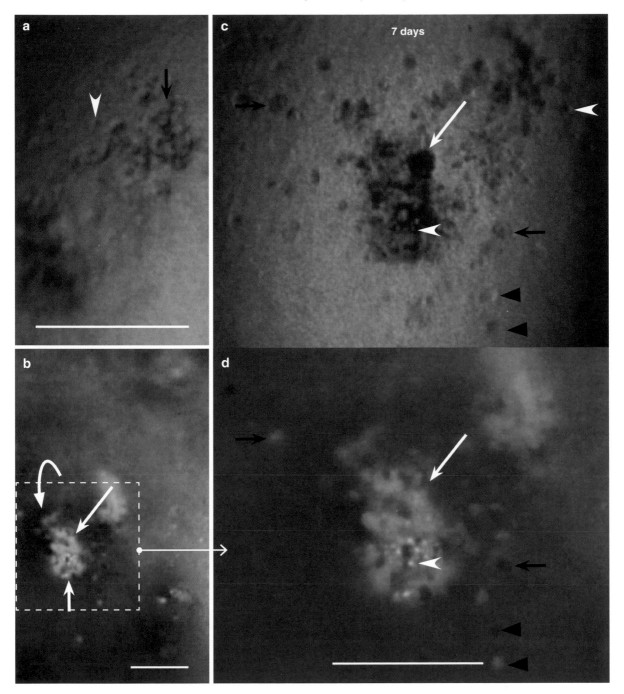

Fig. 2.24 (a) Seven days after symptom onset are visible rounded/abnormal cells, individual (*arrowhead*) or grouped (*arrow*). (b) Survey showing circumscript green staining (*short arrow*) of epithelial infiltrates (*long arrow*) and adjacent surface elevations (dark; *bowed arrow*). The area in frame is shown at higher magnification in (c) and (d). (c) The lesion (*arrow*) contains accumulated rounded/abnormal cells (*white arrowhead*) apparently mixed with cell debris. Rounded/abnormal cells, individual (*white arrowhead*) or grouped (*black arrows*) and cyst-like structures (*black arrowheads*) are visible in the surroundings. (d) Some groups of rounded/abnormal cells (*black arrows*) and some cyst-like structures (*black arrowheads*) stain brilliantly green, others are protruding (*dark*) in the green stained tear film. (In c and d, the arrows and the black arrowheads are placed in corresponding locations)

Nosocomial Infection in Corneal Erosion (Case 10, cont.)

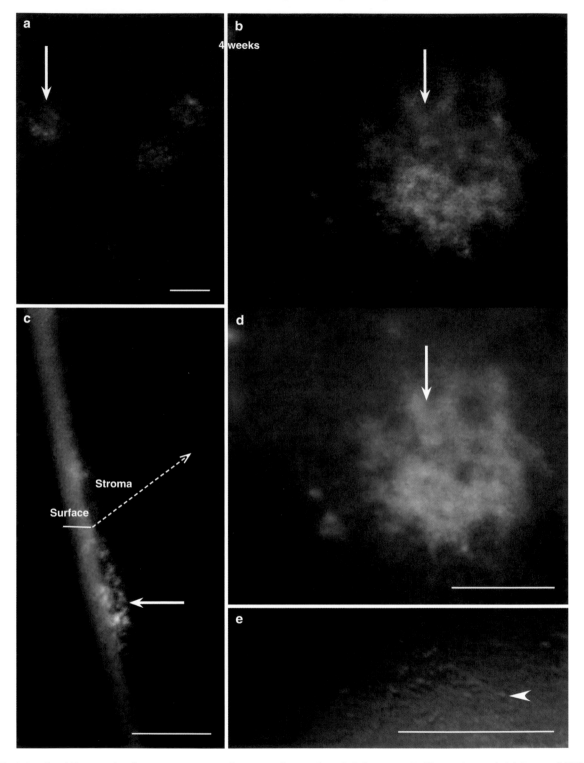

Fig. 2.25 (a–e) Four weeks after symptom onset, the cornea shows subepithelial opacities/infiltrates (*arrows*). (a) Survey. (b) The infiltrate (*arrow*) consists of more or less light-reflecting areas, has indistinct edges, (c) is superficially located below (c, d) an apparently intact surface, and (e) contains rounded/abnormal cells (*arrowhead*). (The arrows in b and d are placed in corresponding locations)

Nosocomial Infection in Corneal Erosion (Case 10, cont.)

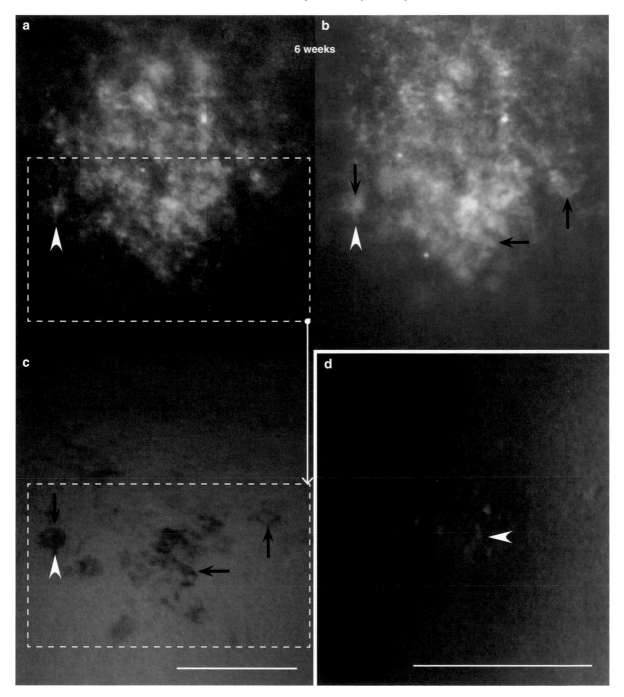

Fig. 2.26 (a–d) Six weeks after symptom onset. (a) A subepithelial opacity/infiltrate with indistinct edges. (b) With fluorescein, the overlying epithelium appears intact. (c) The light-reflecting areas show rounded/abnormal cells (*arrowhead*); the cells seem mixed with light-reflecting material suggestive of cell debris. (The markers are placed in corresponding locations.) (d) A different area showing the presence of grouped rounded/abnormal cells (*arrowhead*)

Nosocomial Infection in Corneal Erosion (Case 10, cont.)

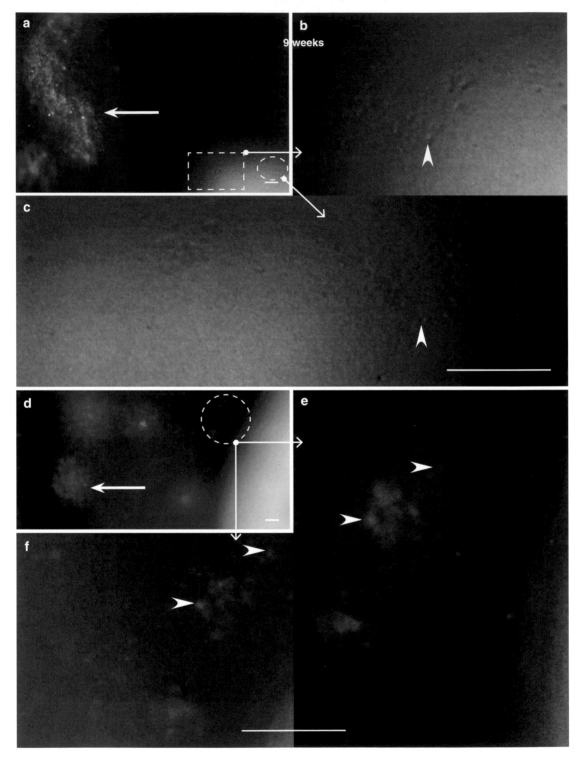

Fig. 2.27 (**a–f**) Nine weeks after symptom onset, the cornea shows (**a** and **d**) many subepithelial opacities/infiltrates (*arrows*) located below (**d**) an apparently intact surface. (**b, c**) show at higher magnification the areas indicated by *frames* in (**a**); rounded/abnormal cells are visible in both (*arrowheads*). (**e, f**) show at higher magnification the area indicated by *frame* in (**d**). In (**f**) are visible groups of rounded/abnormal cells (*arrowheads*), in places possibly mixed with cell debris (*arrow*), and in (**e**) their light-reflecting property. (The markers are placed in corresponding locations)

Nosocomial Infection in Corneal Erosion (Case 10, cont.)

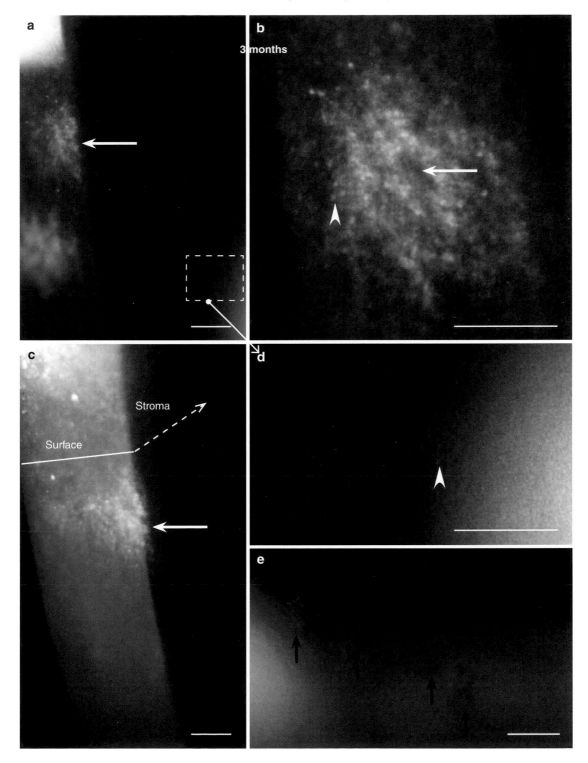

Fig. 2.28 (a–e) Three months after symptom onset. (a, b) The subepithelial opacities/infiltrates (*arrows*) contain (b) light-reflecting dots (*arrowhead*). (c) Shows their location below an apparently intact surface, (d) the presence of rounded/abnormal cells (*arrowhead*) in the area indicated by *frame* in (a), and (e) groups of rounded/abnormal cells (*arrows*). (The arrows in a and b are placed in corresponding locations)

Nosocomial Infection in Corneal Erosion (Case 10, cont.)

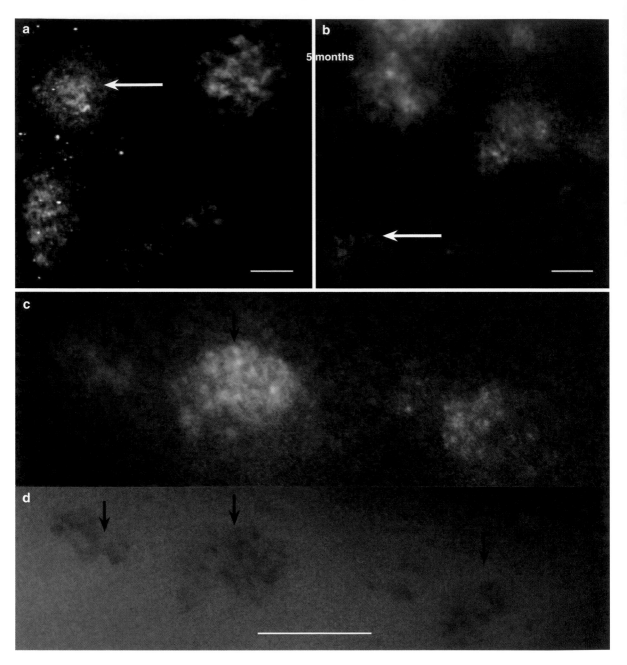

Fig. 2.29 (a–d) Five months after symptom onset, the cornea shows (a, b) subepithelial opacities/infiltrates (*arrows*). In (c, d) are visible groups (*arrows*) of rounded/abnormal cells. (The arrows in c and d are placed in corresponding locations)

Nosocomial Infection in Corneal Erosion (Case 10, cont.)

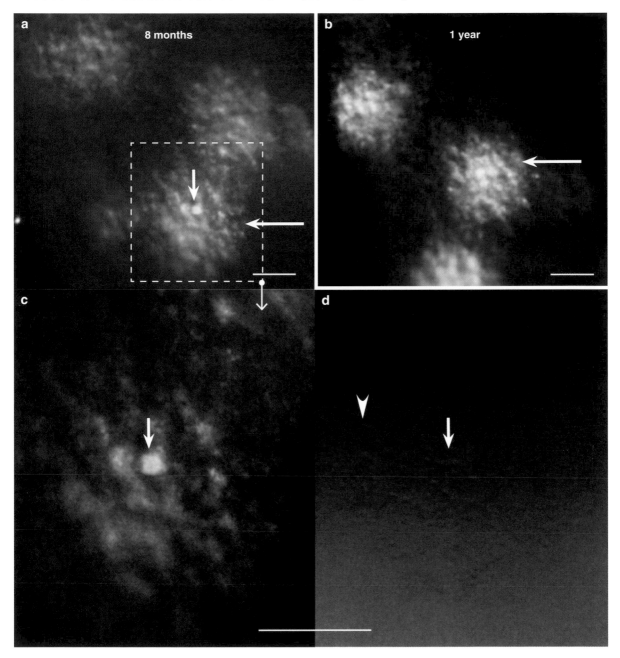

Fig. 2.30 (a–d) The appearance of subepithelial opacities/infiltrates (*long arrows*) (a, c, and d) 8 months and (b) 1 year after the onset of symptoms. The infiltrate indicated by *short arrow* in (a) is shown at higher magnification in (c, d). (c) Fluorescein visualizes a small surface disruption (*arrow*). (d) The infiltrate contains rounded/abnormal cells (*arrowhead*). (The short arrows in a, c, and d are placed in corresponding locations)

Adenovirus Epithelial Keratitis Caused by Various Serotypes (Ad3, 4, and 7)

3

Of the seven patients included in this chapter, each represents a bit of clinical reality with differential diagnostic considerations. In six of them, the infection was verified by virological laboratory. In the last one (Case 7), the diagnosis was clinical, based on findings and a knowledge of a close relative with a verified adenovirus infection. Intrafamilial spread occurred also in cases 2 and 3.

In Case 1, Ad8 infection was considered because of a history of a recent journey to a region where Ad8 is endemic, but the tests showed Ad3.

In Case 2, a combination of red eye and general symptoms implied pharyngoconjunctival fever, but a primary HSV infection, often not thought of at the patient's age because rare, could have given similar initial symptoms; a careful observation of the morphology revealed the true cause.

Severe general symptoms are of serious concern to the parents (daughter in Case 3) and may even result in hospital admission (Case 4); in the latter patient, the combination with red eye was an important diagnostic clue.

Cases 3 and 5 show that coarse epithelial lesions in white eye, which is a typical feature of Thygeson's keratitis, may be seen also in adenovirus-caused keratitis. The common error of diagnosing Thygeson's keratitis as adenovirus is well known; one might wonder if also the converse might occur.

Sometimes, the distribution of changes in adenovirus epithelial keratitis may remind of a branching figure (Case 6) and be interpreted as an HSV dendrite; the differential diagnosis, however, should not be difficult because the substructures of the two substantially differ from each other.

As in Chap. 1 and 2, the time indications given are related to the onset of symptoms as reported by the patients.

H.M. Tabery, *Adenovirus Epithelial Keratitis and Thygeson's Superficial Punctate Keratitis*,
DOI 10.1007/978-3-642-21634-3_3, © Springer-Verlag Berlin Heidelberg 2012

Case 1: Adenovirus: Which Serotype?

Case Report

A 52-year-old woman was treated elsewhere with topical and general antibiotics and with topical acyclovir for keratoconjunctivitis of unknown origin. The symptoms had started shortly after her return from South East Asia. At presentation, 13 days after symptom onset, the right eye was moderately injected, and the corneal epithelium showed many epithelial dots and small opacities. The lids of the left eye were swollen, the conjunctiva showed chemosis and a pseudomembrane in the lower fornix, and the cornea many epithelial dots, several smaller epithelial infiltrates, and a large one; additionally, there were folds of the Descemet's membrane and a mild anterior uveitis. Because possibly exposed to the virus during the journey, Ad8 was considered but serum neutralization test revealed Ad3. In the left cornea developed many subepithelial infiltrates causing decrease in vision. Seven months later she developed a mild anterior uveitis in the left eye; subepithelial infiltrates were still present. Two years after the acute disease, she had episodes of recurrent erosions in the right eye, and also the left eye showed changes (cysts) compatible with recurrent erosion syndrome; at that occasion, all subepithelial infiltrates were gone.

The photographs of the left cornea were taken 13 days, 3 weeks, and 2 months after symptom onset.

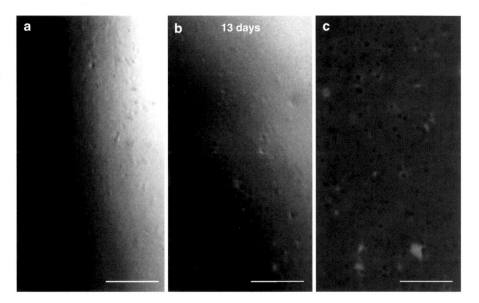

Fig. 3.1 Survey of corneal epithelial changes in Ad3 infection captured 13 days after symptom onset. It shows (**a**, **b**) many dots and (**b**, **c**) many dark spots in the tear film stained green with fluorescein. Fig. 3.3 (*opposite page*) shows some details of the same cornea

Fig. 3.2 Conventional slit lamp photograph of subepithelial opacities/infiltrates, 10 months after the onset of symptoms

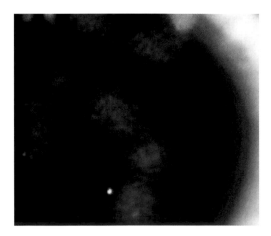

Adenovirus: Which Serotype? (Case 1, cont.)

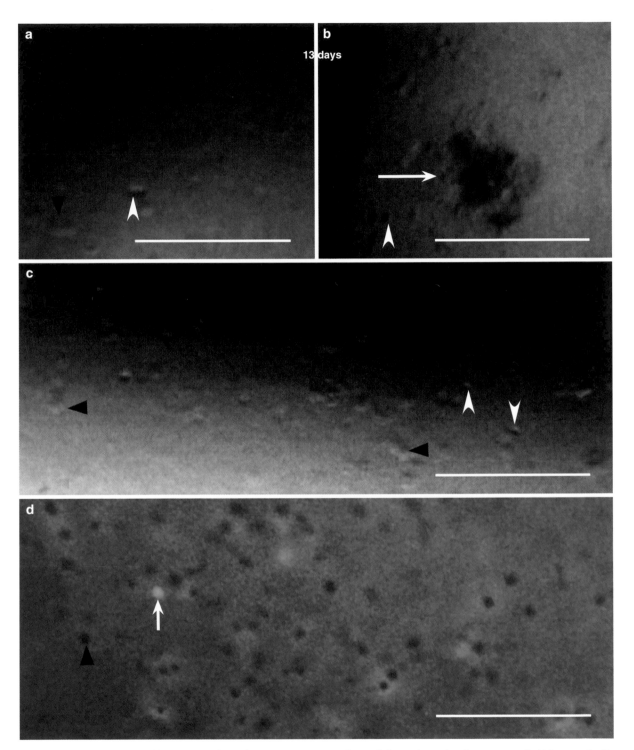

Fig. 3.3 (a–d) Ad3 epithelial keratitis, 13 days after symptom onset. The epithelium shows (a–c) many rounded/abnormal cells (*white arrowheads*), (b) an epithelial infiltrate (*arrow*), and cyst-like structures (*black arrowheads*). (d) shows cyst-like structures protruding (dark; *arrowhead*) in the tear film stained green with fluorescein and a few brilliantly green dots (*arrow*)

Adenovirus: Which Serotype? (Case 1, cont.)

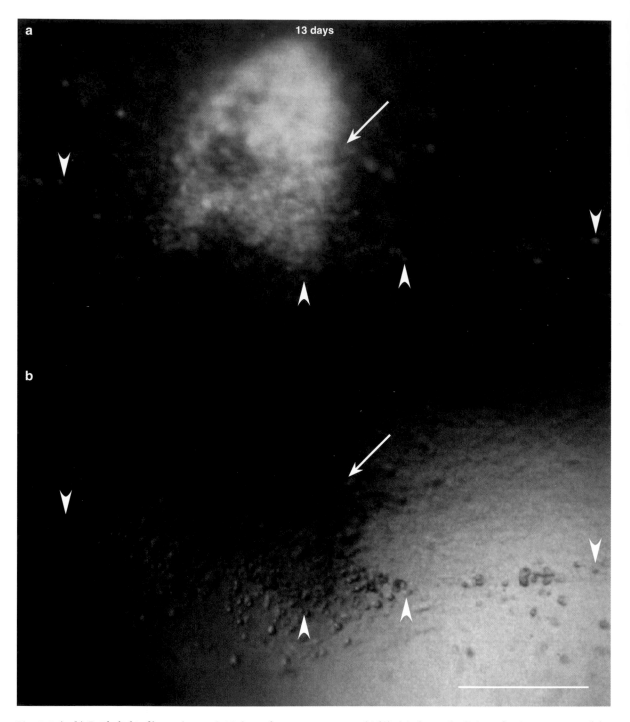

Fig. 3.4 (**a, b**) Epithelial infiltrate (*arrows*) 13 days after symptom onset (Ad3). (**a**) shows the light-reflecting property of the infiltrate and of the rounded/abnormal cells (*arrowheads*). In (**b**) are visible many rounded/abnormal cells (*arrowheads*) at the edges of the lesion and in the surroundings; within the lesion, they are more difficult to discern because they heaped-up and possibly mixed with cell debris. (The markers are placed in corresponding locations)

Adenovirus: Which Serotype? (Case 1, cont.)

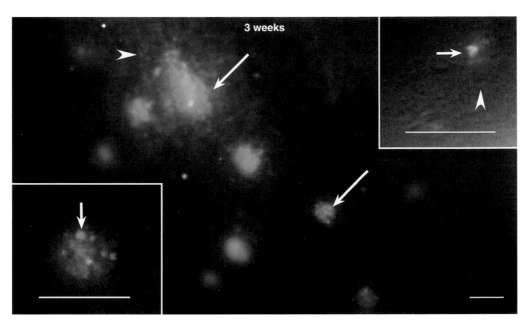

Fig. 3.5 Three weeks after symptom onset (Ad3). The survey shows green fluorescein staining of epithelial infiltrates (*arrows*) and many light-reflecting dots (*arrowhead*) in the surroundings. *Inset (left)*: small green stained dots (*arrow*) within an infiltrate. *Inset (right)*: a green stained dot (*arrow*) and rounded/abnormal cells (*arrowhead*)

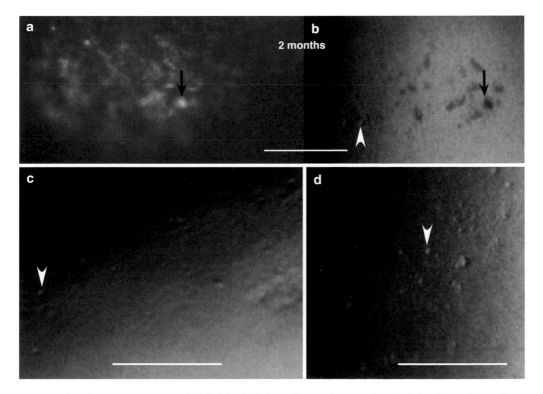

Fig. 3.6 Two months after symptom onset (Ad3). (**a**) The light-reflecting lesion/subepithelial infiltrate has indistinct edges. The *arrow* indicates a location corresponding to that visible in (**b**) as a dense spot (*arrow*). The *arrowhead* points to a rounded/abnormal cell. (**c** and **d**) Rounded/abnormal cells (*arrowheads*) spread in the in-between areas

Case 2: Pharyngoconjunctival Fever

Case Report

A 62-year-old man with redness of the left eye, swollen preauricular lymph node, sore throat, and fever for a week. The right eye was slightly injected. The lids of the left eye were swollen, the conjunctiva injected, and the cornea showed many dot-like surface elevations and a few dots staining green with fluorescein. Six days later, both eyes were injected and showed several epithelial infiltrates, more numerous on the left side. In the meantime, the patient's wife developed the same symptoms. Adenovirus type 3 was identified as the cause. The photographs of the left cornea were taken 13 days after symptom onset.

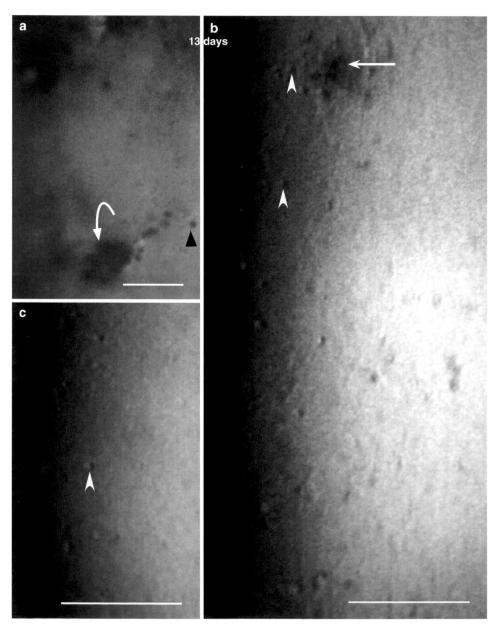

Fig. 3.7 (a–c) Thirteen days after symptom onset (Ad3). The cornea shows (a) larger (*arrow*) and smaller (*arrowhead*) surface elevations (dark in the green stained tear film); (b) an epithelial infiltrate (*arrow*), cyst-like structures (*black arrowhead*); and (b and c) many rounded/abnormal cells (*white arrowheads*)

Case 3: Adenovirus Type 7 in a Contact Lens Wearer and Her Family

Case Report

In this 29-year-old woman, the disease started with redness and irritation in the right eye; the fellow eye became affected 5 days later. The symptoms had subsided but for a slight irritation in the left eye. She presented partly because she was a contact lens wearer, and partly because also her daughter and her husband had developed eye symptoms. At presentation, both eyes were white but the left cornea showed two epithelial infiltrates. A week later, all findings were gone.

The patient's 5-year-old daughter had had fever, sore throat, and pain in the left ear for a week. The right eye was white. The left eye showed a moderate lid swelling, a severe conjunctival injection, conjunctival hemorrhages and erosions, and follicular hyperplasia; the left preauricular lymph node was swollen and tender. A week later, all that was left was only a slight lid swelling and a slight conjunctival injection.

Adenovirus type 7 was found in conjunctival swab performed in the daughter.

The photograph shows the left cornea of the mother, 10 days after the onset of symptoms.

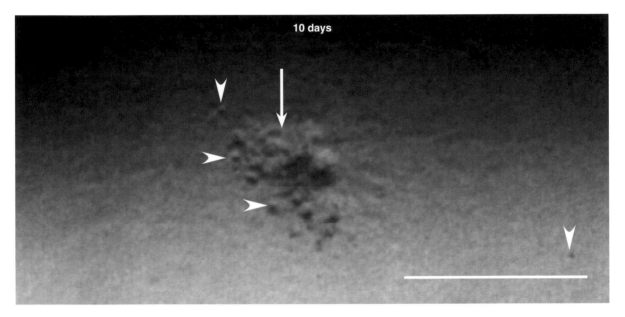

Fig. 3.8 An epithelial infiltrate (*arrow*) showing heaped-up rounded/abnormal cells (*arrowheads*), captured 10 days after the onset of symptoms (Ad7). Rounded/abnormal cells are visible also outside the lesion (*arrowheads*)

Comment

It is more common that small children become infected in nursery school or kindergarten and transmit the infection to their parents, but in this case it seemed to have been the other way round.

In a white eye, lesions such as that shown in Fig. 3.8 are suggestive of Thygeson's keratitis. The clue is the patient's history.

Case 4: Red Eye: A Diagnostic Clue

Case Report

A 36-year-old man was admitted to the Infection Clinic because of general symptoms. In combination with red eyes, adenovirus was suspected and later identified as type 3. Eight days after onset, both eyes were injected and the corneae showed many epithelial infiltrates that were still present two weeks later. The patient's preschool children had had a "cold."

The photographs of the left cornea were taken 22 days after the onset of symptoms.

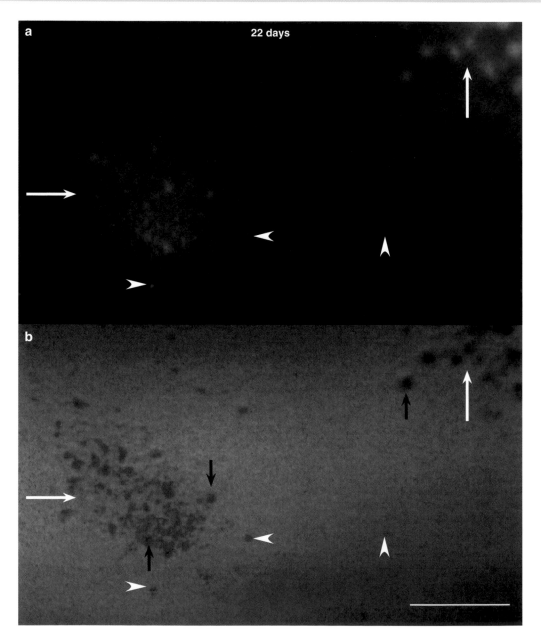

Fig. 3.9 (a, b) Twenty-two days after symptom onset (Ad3): (a) lesions (*white arrows*) lacking defined edges show light-reflecting spots (*black arrows*) and dots (*arrowheads*). In (b) it is visible that the light-reflecting appearance is partly caused by clumps of material (*black arrows*), probably cell debris; discernible rounded/abnormal cells are indicated by *arrowheads*. (The markers are placed in corresponding locations.) Cf. Fig. 3.10 (*opposite page*)

Case 5: Adenovirus or Thygeson's Keratitis?

Case Report

A 35-year-old woman with irritation in both eyes for 3 days had a bilateral follicular conjunctivitis caused by adenovirus type 4. Eighteen days after the onset of symptoms, she presented again because of she could not see clearly. Both eyes were white but the corneae showed many epithelial infiltrates.

The photographs of the right cornea were taken 18 days after the onset of symptoms.

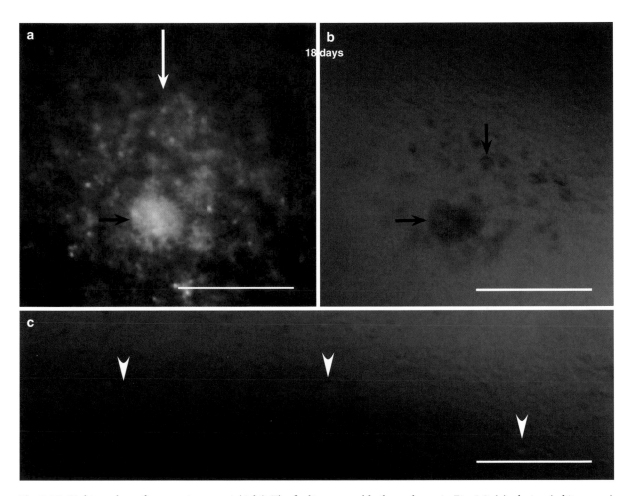

Fig. 3.10 Eighteen days after symptom onset (Ad4). The findings resemble those shown in Fig. 3.9: (**a**) a lesion (*white arrow*) lacking defined edges and composed of light-reflecting spots (*black arrow*) and dots; (**b**) clumps of material (*arrows*) suggestive of cell debris; (**c**) individual rounded/abnormal cells (*arrowheads*) spread in an in-between area

Comment

Similarly to case 3, in a white eye showing coarse epithelial lesions (infiltrates) the patient's history is important for differentiation between adenovirus and Thygeson's keratitis. In this case, the specimen for virological tests was taken early during the conjunctival stage.

Case 6: Adenovirus or HSV Epithelial Keratitis?

Case Report

A 73-year-old man with irritation and redness in the right eye. The duration of symptoms was one week. The right eye was injected, and the cornea showed branching figures reminiscent of HSV. The epithelium healed within 10 days. Virus isolation test showed adenovirus; serotyping was not done.

   The photographs of the right cornea were taken one week after symptom onset.

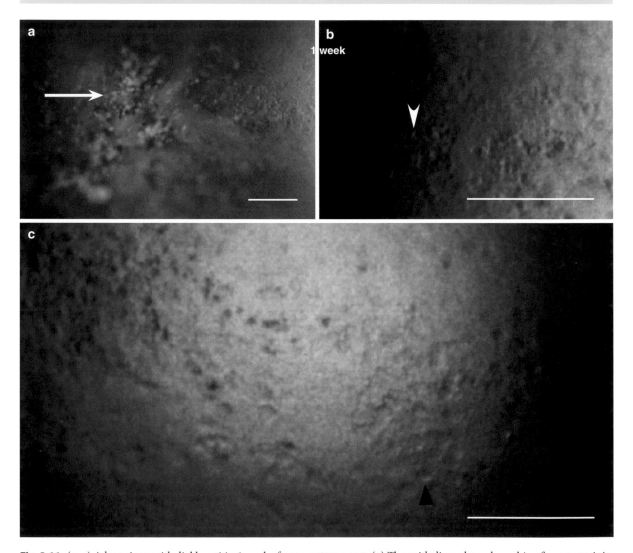

Fig. 3.11 (a–c) Adenovirus epithelial keratitis, 1 week after symptom onset. (a) The epithelium shows branching figures reminiscent of HSV dendritic keratitis. The resemblance is only superficial. The substructure shows features compatible with adenovirus infection: (b) rounded/abnormal cells (*white arrowhead*) and (c) many cyst-like structures (*black arrowhead*)

Fig. 3.12 (a–c) (*Opposite page*) Adenovirus epithelial keratitis. One week after symptom onset, the cornea shows many epithelial infiltrates (*straight arrows*) which (a) are light-reflecting, (b) have granular appearance, and (c) show a circumscript green fluorescein staining and adjacent surface elevations (dark; *bowed arrow*). In all photographs are visible rounded/abnormal cells (*white arrowheads*) and in (b) also cyst-like structures (*black arrowhead*). (The straight arrows are placed in corresponding locations)

Case 7: Adenovirus Infection: A Clinical Diagnosis

Case Report

A 42-year-old woman, whose sister had a proven adenovirus infection, was seen a week after the onset of symptoms. Both eyes were injected and the left cornea showed several epithelial infiltrates. The diagnosis was clinical.

The photographs of the left cornea were taken one week after symptom onset.

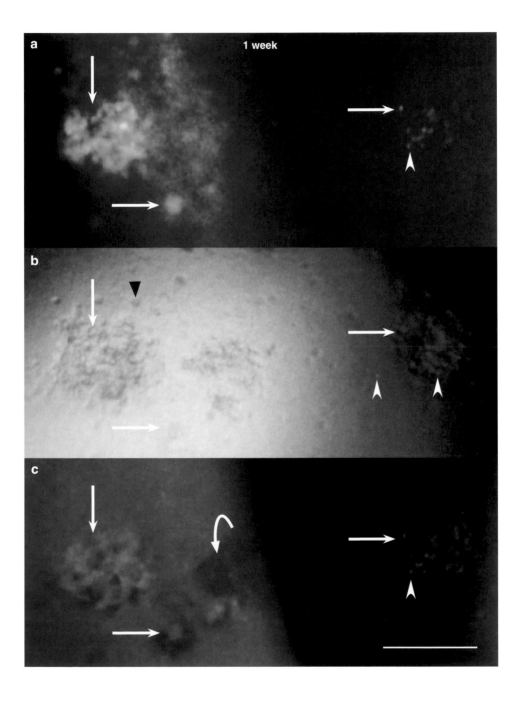

The Development of Subepithelial Infiltrates: A Sequence of Events

4

The preceding chapters show the appearance of subepithelial infiltrates following infections with various adenovirus serotypes captured in different patients at various points of time. This chapter features a sequence of events occurring in the same corneal area in a patient infected with adenovirus type 8 (Ad8) during a nosocomial outbreak. The series starts 3 weeks after symptom onset and ends 3 years later.

A *visualization* in detail of a sequence of events occurring in the same corneal area is not an easy undertaking. To perform this task to perfection in a living, moving human eye is difficult, mainly because there are no reference points except the changes themselves; they are not an ideal substitute because changing between occasions, but that is all there is. In the present series, the cornea was heavily affected but there was an area that could be recognized for as long as 15 months. After its pattern had dissipated, the exact orientation was lost. Hence, the series ends with changes captured either in the same location or very close to it.

As previously mentioned (Chap. 2), *subepithelial opacities/infiltrates* are considered to be a sequela of adenovirus infections, and the clinical watershed seems to be the moment when the corneal surface appears restored, as far as can be judged by an absence of fluorescein staining. When exactly the subepithelial stroma becomes involved, early after symptom onset or later on, is unclear. The rounded/abnormal cells per se are no reliable indicators partly because they appear early after symptom onset, and partly because in the living human cornea their exact position in depth versus the epithelial basement membrane cannot be estimated in two-dimensional images. The only phenomenon indicating subepithelial involvement is the second component of the infiltrates, i.e., the superficially located light-reflecting structures morphologically compatible with a disturbance of the fine lamellar organization of the corneal stroma. It is probable, however, that initial changes escape detection.

As both the cellular and the stromal components are light-reflecting, in areas where both are present the rounded/abnormal cells may be difficult or impossible to identify in focal illumination. Fortunately, the two components can be optically separated from each other using retroillumination; a comparison of photographs capturing the same area in both illumination modes reveals their respective representations in the infiltrates. In the present series, the *cellular component* diminished with time. After 16 weeks, its distribution pattern could no longer be compared between occasions, but the rounded/abnormal cells did not disappear entirely; some were still present 3 years after symptom onset. The events occurring in the *stromal component* were more difficult to judge because even small changes of illumination angles caused by the inevitable eye movements may result in a false impression of more or less pronounced changes; the trend was toward a slow expansion for several months, and a slow regress starting about a year after symptom onset. In some photographs, the same structures could be discerned in photographs taken 2 weeks (Figs. 4.15 and 4.17) and 1 month (Figs. 4.19 and 4.21) apart.

Accompanying *secondary phenomena* were few: surface elevations, focal surface disruptions (rare), and small dark/light-reflecting spots implying a contribution of cell debris.

Case Report

The patient was a 45-year-old woman examined in the Emergency Department because of foreign body sensation in the right eye. The superior conjunctiva showed a small erosion but no subtarsal foreign body was found, and her symptoms subsided rapidly. A week later she woke up with a red right eye. The lids were swollen, the conjunctiva injected, and the lower fornix showed follicular hyperplasia. The left eye was white. Adenovirus was suspected. Two days later, the right cornea appeared dusty. After a further week, both eyes were injected and both corneae showed many epithelial infiltrates. Three weeks after symptom onset she was symptom-free except for hazy vision in both eyes. Her visual acuity fluctuated, slowly ameliorated, and returned to normal 4 months after symptom onset. After that, she had no problems despite many subepithelial opacities/infiltrates that had developed in both eyes and partly involved the central cornea.

The photographs were taken in the paracentral nasal area of the more severely affected right eye.

H.M. Tabery, *Adenovirus Epithelial Keratitis and Thygeson's Superficial Punctate Keratitis*, DOI 10.1007/978-3-642-21634-3_4, © Springer-Verlag Berlin Heidelberg 2012

Survey 1

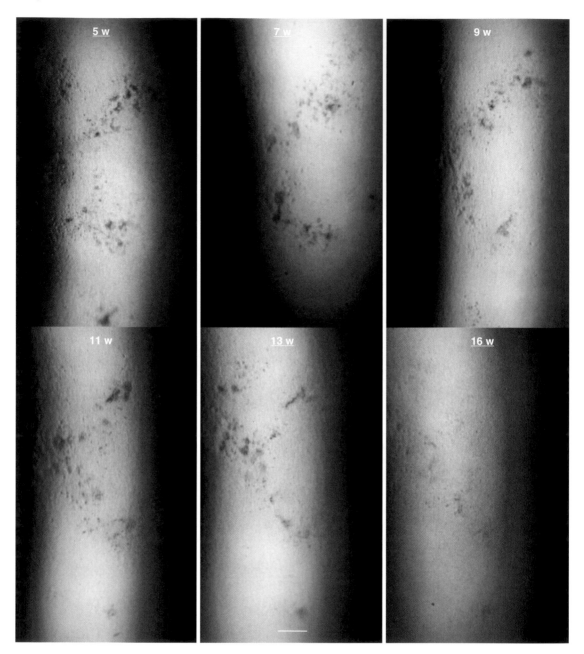

Fig. 4.1 Survey of development occurring in the same corneal area between 5 and 16 weeks after symptom onset. This series visualizes changes in distribution of the rounded/abnormal cells. In the absence of reference points other than the changes itself, exact locations cannot be pin-pointed but the shape of the figure allows comparisons between the occasions; later on, a comparable distribution pattern was no longer detectable. The light-reflecting property of the lesions captured at 5,7,13 and 16 weeks (underlined) is shown in Fig. 4.2 (*opposite page*)

Details captured at successive occasions, starting 3 weeks after symptom onset, are shown in Figs. 4.3–4.30, and further development in Figs. 4.31–4.36.

Survey 2

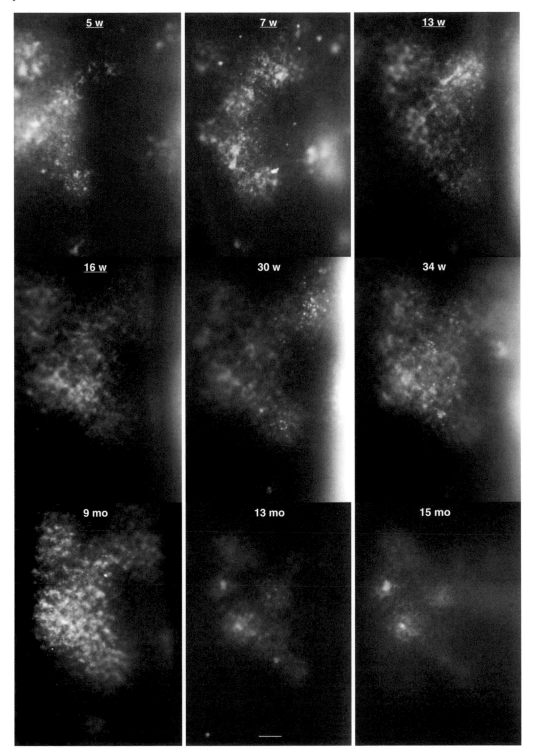

Fig. 4.2 Survey of development occurring in the same corneal area between 5 weeks and 15 months after symptom onset. This series visualizes light-reflecting changes, a property shared by the rounded/abnormal cells and changes in the superficial stroma. As in Fig. 4.1, exact locations cannot be pin-pointed but the shape of the figure is recognizable up to 15 months

3 Weeks After Onset

Fig. 4.3 (a, b) Survey, 3 weeks after symptom onset. Visible are many light-reflecting rounded/abnormal cells, individual (*arrowheads*) and grouped (*arrows*). The area indicated by *frame* is shown at higher magnification in Fig. 4.4a, below. (The markers are placed in corresponding locations; b is a composed photograph)

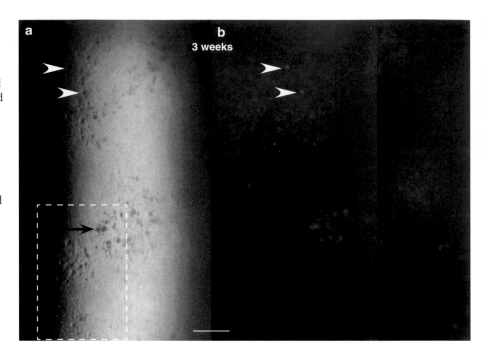

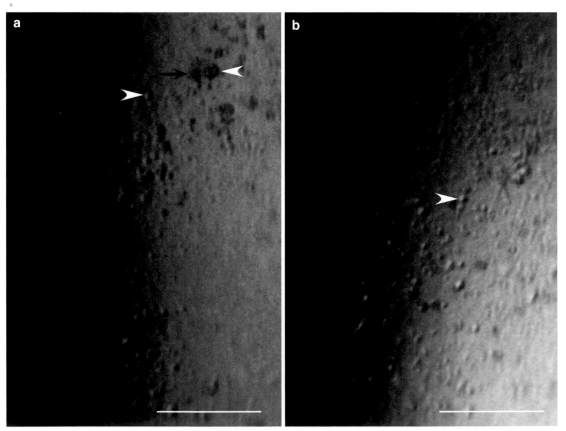

Fig. 4.4 (a) In the area indicated by frame in Fig. 4.3a are visible many rounded/abnormal cells, individual (*arrowhead*) and grouped, some located within darker spots (*arrow*). (b) A different area showing many rounded/abnormal cells (*arrowhead*)

4 Weeks After Onset

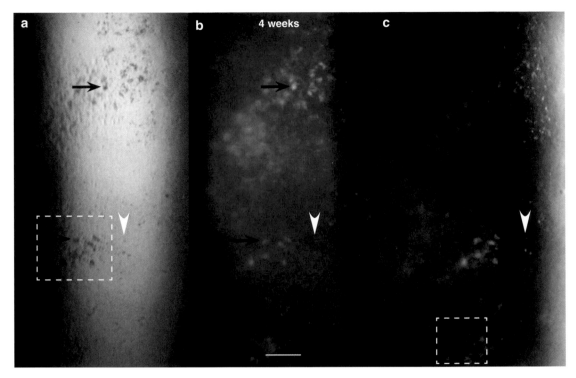

Fig. 4.5 (a–c) Survey, 4 weeks after symptom onset. With fluorescein (c) it is visible that the rounded/abnormal cells, both individual (*arrowheads*) or grouped (*arrows*), are located below intact surface layer/s. The area in *frame* in (a) is shown at higher magnification in Fig. 4.6a and in (c) in Fig. 4.6b (below). (The markers are placed in corresponding locations)

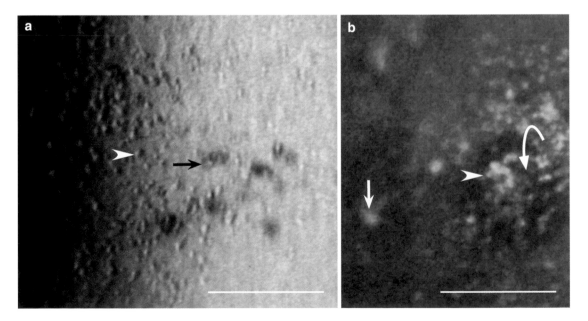

Fig. 4.6 (a) Many rounded/abnormal cells (*arrowhead*) within the area indicated by frame in Fig. 4.5a; some are located within darker spots (*arrow*). (b) In the area indicated by frame in Fig. 4.5c are visible heaped-up rounded/abnormal cells (*arrowhead*) in areas of surface elevation (dark in the green stained tear film, *bowed arrow*) and a few green dots (*straight arrow*)

5 Weeks After Onset

Fig. 4.7 (a, b) Survey, 5 weeks after symptom onset. The cellular component (*arrows*) is still pronounced. The areas within *frames* are shown at higher magnification in Fig. 4.8 (below): the *oval* frame in (a), the *white rectangular* frame in (b), and the *black rectangular* one in (c). (The arrows are placed in corresponding locations)

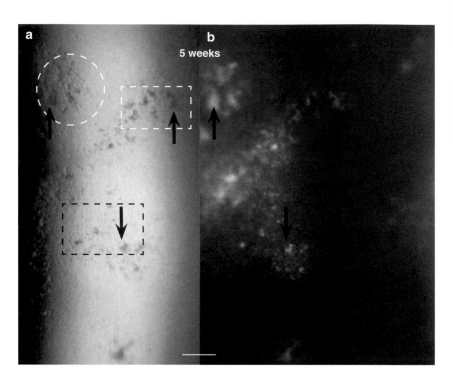

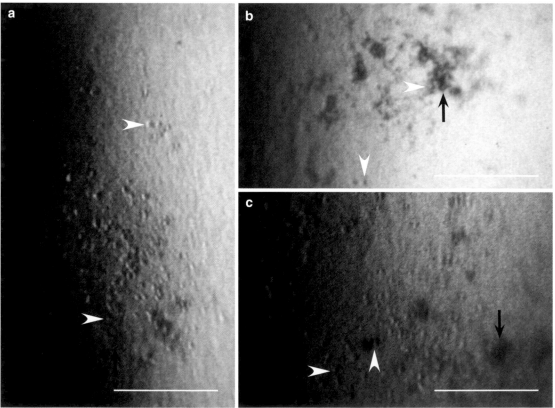

Fig. 4.8 (a–c) In all the three areas indicated by frames in Fig. 4.7 many rounded/abnormal cells (*arrowheads*) are visible. They are more difficult to discern within the dark spots (*arrows*)

7 Weeks After Onset

Fig. 4.9 (a–c) Survey, 7 weeks after symptom onset. (a, b) The cellular component (*arrows*), (c) located below a preserved surface layer, causes surface elevations (dark in the green stained tear film). The area indicated by *frame* is shown in Fig. 4.10 (below). (The arrows are placed in corresponding locations)

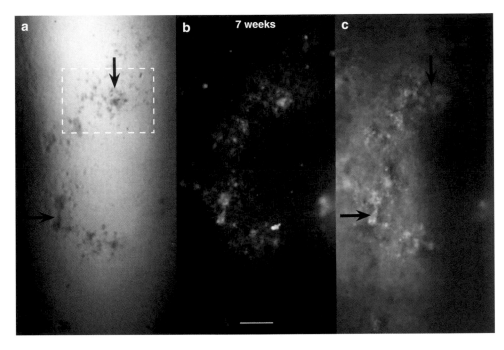

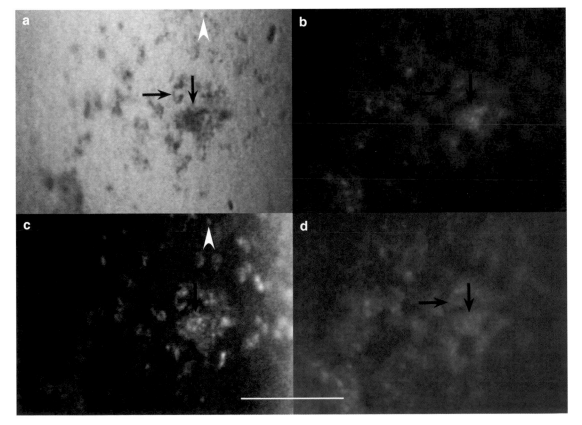

Fig. 4.10 (a–d) The area indicated by frame in Fig. 4.9 a shows, similarly to Fig. 4.8 (*opposite page*), (a and c) rounded/abnormal cells (*arrowheads*) and (a) dark spots (*arrows*) that (b–d) are strongly light-reflecting. (d) The epithelial surface is preserved. (The markers are placed in corresponding locations)

11 Weeks After Onset

Fig. 4.11 (a, b) Survey, 11 weeks after symptom onset. (a) As before, there is a propensity to form dark spots (*arrows*). (b) Fluorescein reveals elevations (dark) of a preserved surface layer. Areas indicated by *frames* are shown at higher magnification in Fig. 4.12 (*below*) : *white* rectangular frame in (a), *black* rectangular frame in (b), and *circular* frame in (c) (The *arrows* are placed in corresponding locations)

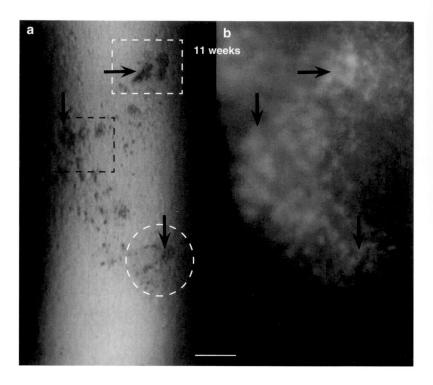

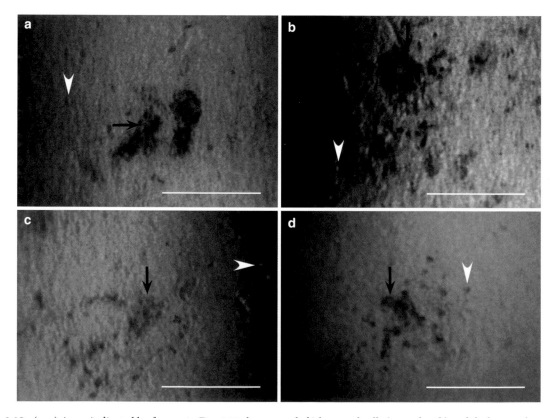

Fig. 4.12 (a–c) Areas indicated by frames in Fig. 4.11 show rounded/abnormal cells (*arrowheads*) and dark spots (*arrows*) in which such cells are more difficult to discern. (d) shows another area with similar features

13 Weeks After Onset

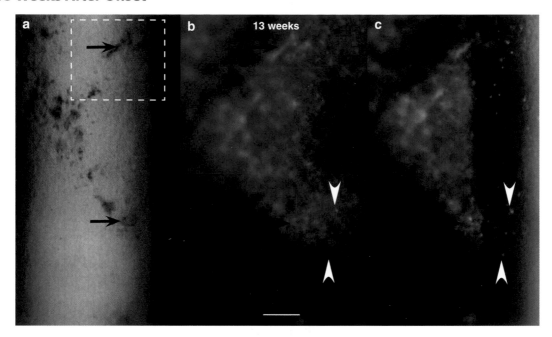

Fig. 4.13 (a–c) Survey, 13 weeks after onset. Visible are (a) dark spots (*arrows*) and (b, c) some individual rounded/abnormal cells (*arrowheads*). The stromal component (b) is now more pronounced. The *area in frame* is shown in Fig. 4.14 a-b (*below*). (The markers are placed in corresponding locations)

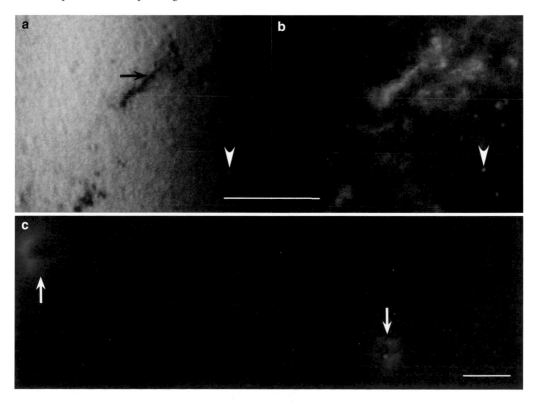

Fig. 4.14 (a and b) show rounded/abnormal cells (*arrowheads*) and (a) dark spots (*arrow*); in (b) their light-reflecting property is visible. (The markers are placed in corresponding locations.) (c) Two small areas of surface disruption (*arrows*) captured at the same occasion. (Fluorescein and blue filter)

16 Weeks After Onset

Fig. 4.15 (a, b) Survey, 16 weeks after symptom onset. (a) shows that the cellular component (*arrows*) has further diminished and (b) the stromal one predominates. The areas indicated by *frames* are shown at higher magnification in Fig. 4.16 (*below*), the in *rectangular* frame in (a and c), and that in *circular* frame in (b). The *arrowhead* indicates an area still recognizable 2 weeks later (cf. Fig. 4.17, *opposite page*). (The arrows are placed in approximately corresponding locations)

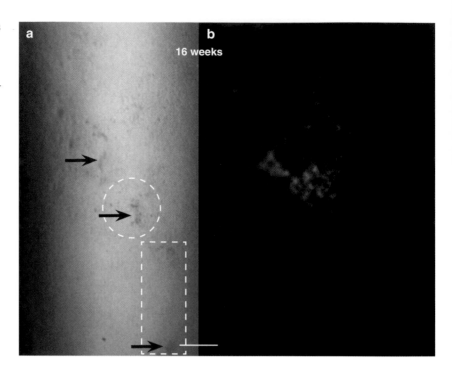

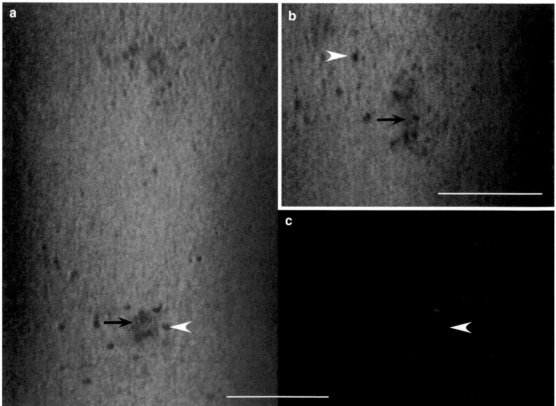

Fig. 4.16 (a–c) The areas indicated (a) by rectangular frame and (b) by circular frame in Fig. 4.15 show small dark spots (*arrows*) and rounded/abnormal cells (*arrowheads*). (c) Shows their light-reflecting property. (The markers in a and c are placed in corresponding locations)

18 Weeks After Onset

Fig. 4.17 (a, b) Survey, 18 weeks after symptom onset. A comparable pattern of rounded/abnormal cells could no longer be found. With fluorescein (b), the surface appears intact. The *arrowhead* indicates the same structure as in Fig. 4.15 (*opposite page*). The *black arrows* in a and b indicate corresponding locations

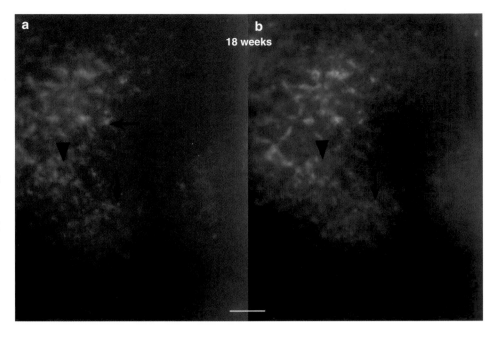

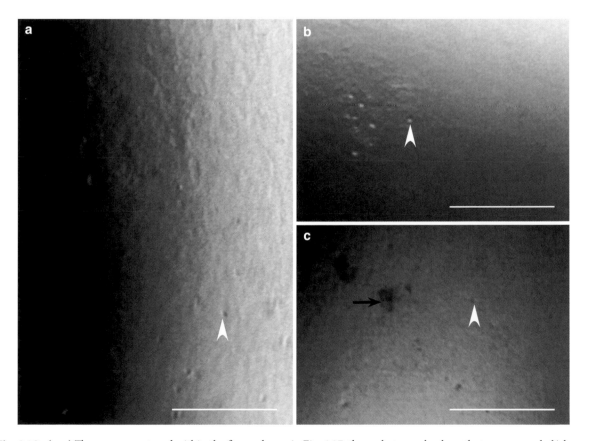

Fig. 4.18 (a–c) Three areas captured within the figure shown in Fig. 4.17; these photographs show that some rounded/abnormal cells (*arrowheads*) and dark spots (c, *arrow*) are still present

5 Months After Onset

Fig. 4.19 (a, b) Survey, 5 months after symptom onset. (a) The majority of the rounded/abnormal cells have disappeared and the figure consists mainly of (b) the stromal component. Although in (a) no figure comparable to that of (b) can be discerned, there are two small areas the location of which can be identified; the area in *white frame* is shown at higher magnification in Fig. 4.20a and that in *black frame* in Fig. 4.20b and c (below). (The arrows are placed in corresponding locations.) The location indicated by *arrowhead* and *circular frame* is still recognizable 1 month later (Fig. 4.21, *opposite page*)

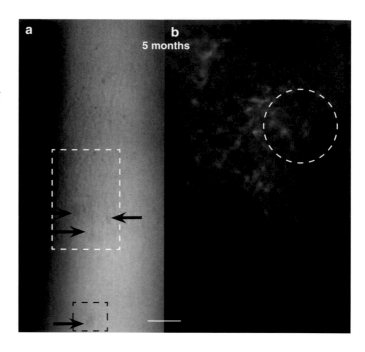

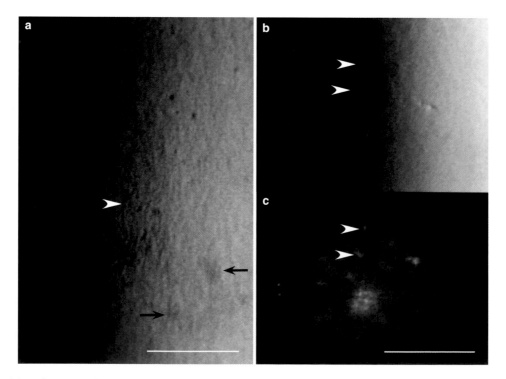

Fig. 4.20 (a) In the area indicated by *white frame* in Fig. 4.19 a a few rounded/abnormal cells (*arrowhead*) and dark spots (*arrows*) are visible. (The *arrows* are placed in the same location as in Fig. 4.19 a.) (b, c) Also the area indicated by *black frame* in Fig. 4.19 a shows rounded/abnormal cells, individual (*arrowheads*) and grouped (*arrows*) (The markers in b and c are placed in corresponding locations)

6 Months After Onset

Fig. 4.21 Survey, 6 months after symptom onset. The area indicated by rectangular *frame* is shown at higher magnification in Fig. 4.22 (below). The *arrowhead* and the *circular frame* indicate the same location as in Fig. 4.19 (*opposite page*). Although a month later, the pattern is still recognizable. (Composed photograph)

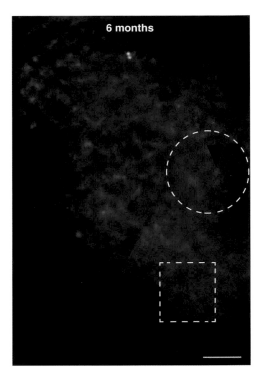

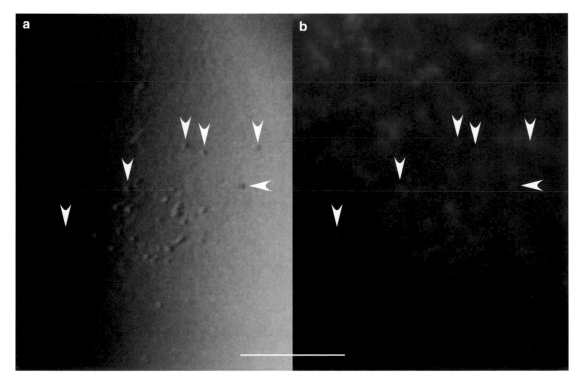

Fig. 4.22 (**a, b**) The area indicated by frame in Fig. 4.21 shows (**a**) rounded/abnormal cells (*arrowheads*) which in (**b**) can be distinguished from their light-reflecting surroundings by comparison of patterns. (The arrowheads are placed in corresponding locations)

7.5 Months After Onset

Fig. 4.23   Survey, 7.5 months after symptom onset. The area indicated by *frame* is shown at higher magnification in Fig. 4.24 (*below*). (The *arrows* indicating two light reflecting spots are placed in locations corresponding to those in Fig. 4.24)

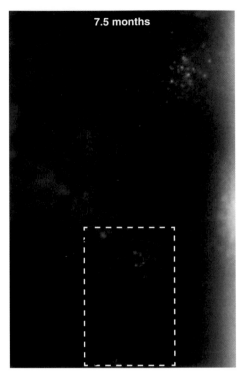

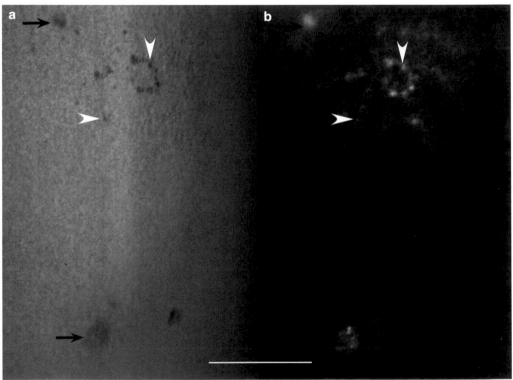

Fig. 4.24   (**a, b**) The area indicated by frame in Fig. 4.23 shows (**a**) rounded/abnormal cells (*arrowheads*) and dark spots (*arrows*); in (**b**) is visible that both are light-reflecting. (The markers are placed in corresponding locations.) Cf. also *opposite page* capturing the same area a month later

8.5 Months After Onset

Fig. 4.25 Survey, 8.5 months after symptom onset. The area indicated by *frame* is shown at higher magnification in Fig. 4.26 (*below*). It is the same area as that shown in Figs. 4.23 and 4.24. (The arrows indicate the same locations as in Fig. 4.26)

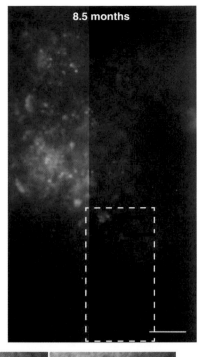

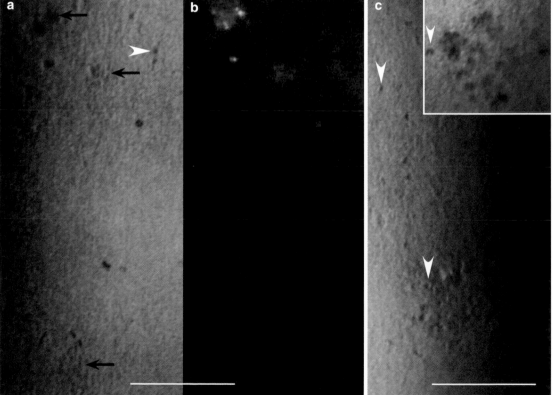

Fig. 4.26 (**a–c**) and *inset*. The area indicated by frame in Fig. 4.25 (the same area as in Fig. 4.24, *opposite page*) shows the same phenomena as before, i.e., (**a**) some rounded/abnormal cells (*arrowhead*) and dark spots (*arrows*) that (**b**) are light-reflecting. (**c**) and inset shows the presence of several rounded/abnormal cells (*arrowheads*), individual or grouped, present in two different areas of the same lesion

9.5 and 11.5 Months After Onset

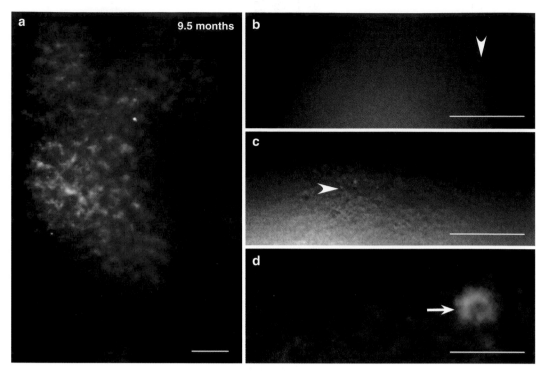

Fig. 4.27 (a) Survey, 9.5 months after symptom onset. (b, c) Rounded/abnormal cells (*arrowheads*) are still present. (d) An area of defect in the epithelial surface (*arrow*) is visualized with fluorescein

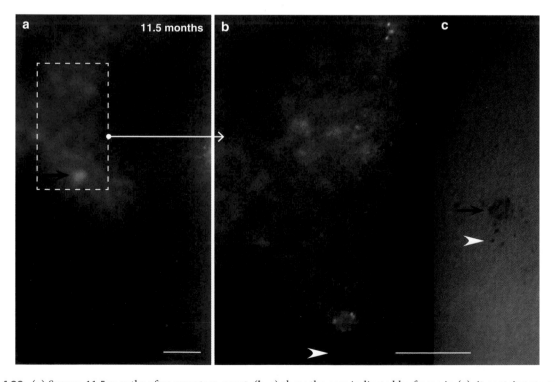

Fig. 4.28 (a) Survey, 11.5 months after symptom onset. (b, c) show the area indicated by frame in (a); it contains rounded/abnormal cells (*arrowheads*) and (a) light-reflecting spots (*arrows*) that in (c) appear dark. (The arrows in a, b and the markers in b, c are placed in corresponding locations)

13 and 15 Months After Onset

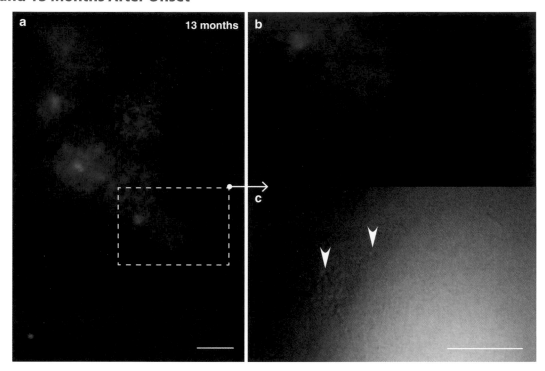

Fig. 4.29 (a) Survey, 13 months after symptom onset. The figure is smaller and starts to separate in individual flecks. (b, c) The area indicated by *frame* in (a) shows (b) light-reflecting spots and (c) a few rounded/abnormal cells (*arrowheads*). (The arrows are placed in corresponding locations)

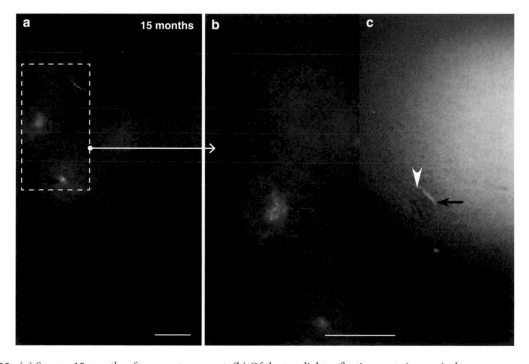

Fig. 4.30 (a) Survey, 15 months after symptom onset. (b) Of the two light-reflecting spots (*arrows*), the upper one contains light-reflecting dots. (c) Grouped rounded/abnormal cells (*arrowhead*) within a spot, probably in the same location as in (b). (The arrows are placed in corresponding locations)

1 Year and 6 Months After Onset

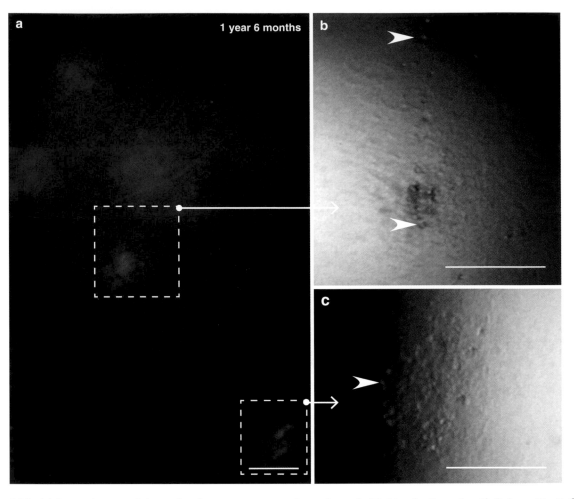

Fig. 4.31 (a) Survey 1 year and 6 months after symptom onset. Several rounded light-reflecting subepithelial opacities/infiltrates in the area previously showing a confluent figure. (b, c) show the presence of rounded/abnormal cells (*arrowheads*), individual or grouped

2 Years and 5 Months After Onset

Fig. 4.32 (a, b) Survey, 2 years and 5 months after symptom onset. (a) Many of the rounded light-reflecting subepithelial opacities/infiltrates contain a strongly light-reflecting spot (*arrows*). (Composed photograph.) (b) With fluorescein, the epithelial surface appears intact but in places elevated (dark; *bowed arrow*). The upper light-reflecting spot seems pigmented. The area in *frame* is shown at higher magnification in Fig. 4.33. (The black arrows are placed in corresponding locations)

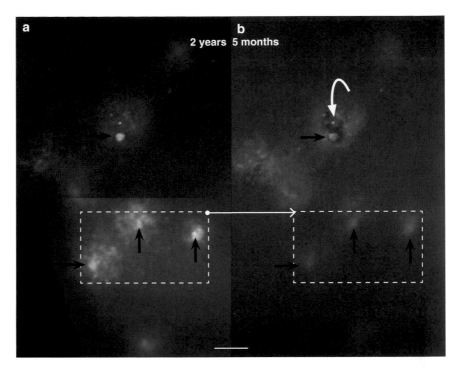

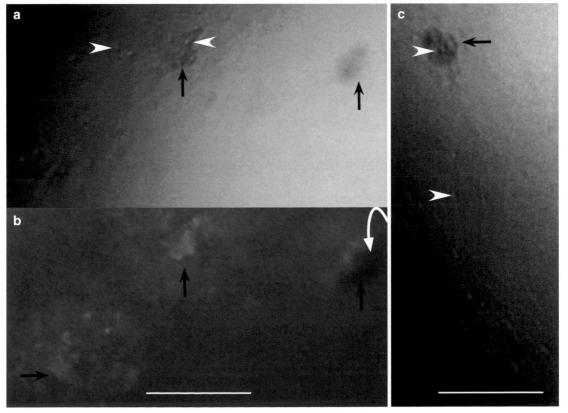

Fig. 4.33 (a–c) The area indicated by frame in Fig. 4.32 shows (a) a few rounded/abnormal cells (*arrowheads*) and dark spots (*arrows*). (b) With fluorescein is visible a surface elevation (dark; *bowed arrow*). (The black arrows are placed in corresponding locations). In (c) is visible another area showing rounded/abnormal cells (*arrowheads*) and a dark spot (*arrow*). For further examples captured at the same occasion see Fig. 4.34 (overleaf)

2 Years and 5 Months After Onset (cont.)

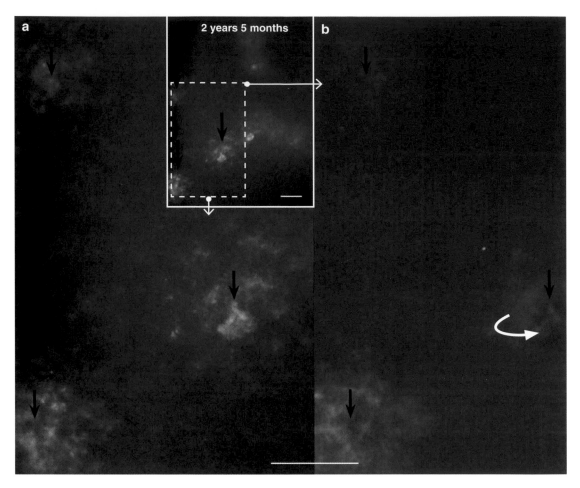

Fig. 4.34 *Inset*: Survey, captured 2 years and 5 months after symptom onset in an area different from that shown in Fig. 4.32; it shows several rounded light-reflecting subepithelial opacities/infiltrates some of which contain a dense light-reflecting spot (*arrows*). The area in *frame* is shown at higher magnification in (**a**) and (**b**). (**a**) The light-reflecting spots (*arrows*) are slightly pigmented (brownish). (**b**) With fluorescein, the surface appears preserved. The *bowed arrow* indicates a surface elevation (dark). (The black arrows are placed in corresponding locations)

2 Years and 8.5 Months, and 3 Years After Onset

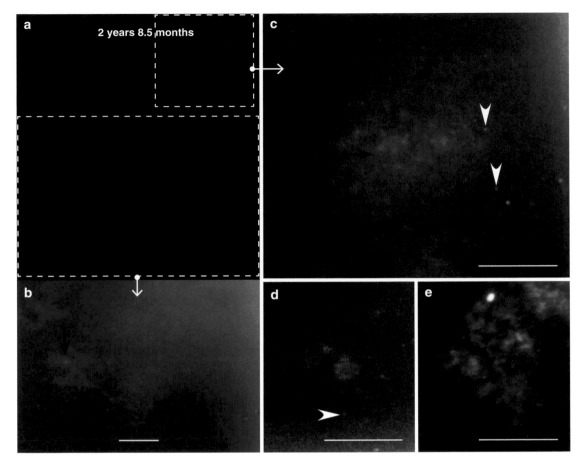

Fig. 4.35 (**a**) Survey, 2 years and 8.5 months after symptom onset. Light-reflecting flecks/subepithelial infiltrates (*arrows*) are still present. (**b**) With fluorescein, the surface appears intact. (The *arrows* are placed in corresponding locations.) (**c**) At the edges of the fleck indicated by *frame* in (**a**) and outside it are visible light-reflecting dots (*arrowheads*) that might represent rounded/abnormal cells. Such cells are clearly visible in (**d**) (*arrowhead*). (**d** and **e**) additionally show spots that appear pigmented (*arrows*)

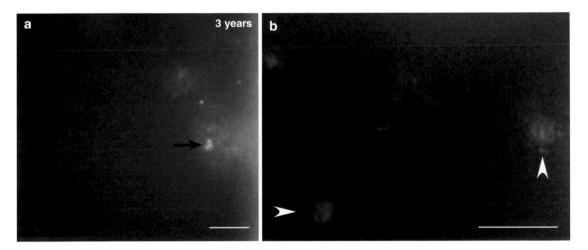

Fig. 4.36 (**a**) Survey, 3 years after symptom onset. Light-reflecting subepithelial opacities/infiltrates are still present; some show a strongly light-reflecting spot (*arrow*). (**b**) Some of the light-reflecting spots seem pigmented (*arrow*); visible are also some rounded/abnormal cells (*arrowheads*)

Part II

Thygeson's Superficial Punctate Keratitis

About Thygeson's Superficial Punctate Keratitis (TSPK)

Since Thygeson's original report in *1950* on 26 patients, over 300 cases have been described in the literature. In *typical* cases, the cornea shows one, a few, or several (20–30) coarse opacities apparently located in the epithelium; occasionally, the changes are diffusely spread with only small aggregates instead of coarse lesions (*atypical* cases). Subepithelial opacities are rare and, if developing, mild and transient (some more severe ones, however, have been reported in the literature). TSPK is basically a bilateral disease, but the manifestations can be unilateral when examined. TSPK *causes* ocular discomfort, irritation, photophobia, tearing, and transitory disturbances of visual acuity. Typically, the eye is white but it might be slightly injected during exacerbations.

TSPK runs a prolonged *course* with numerous exacerbations and remissions, with disease duration reported to range between a month up till 40 years. The duration, however, is difficult to estimate, partly because exacerbations occur even after several symptom-free years, and partly because the keratitis does not always cause symptoms. During long-term follow-ups, I have seen several patients who became symptom-free despite the persistence of epithelial disease, several patients with bilateral disease yet symptoms in one eye only, and a few who denied any symptoms whatsoever (these were patients referred from opticians because of corneal findings, and they were angry because all they wanted were contact lenses).

The *origin* of TSPK is obscure. It occurs in many parts of the world, in both sexes; the youngest reported patient was 2.5 years and the eldest, reported in this volume, 81 years old. TSPK seems neither contagious, nor associated with systemic diseases and, so far, no infectious agent has been identified as its regular cause. A significant association between TSPK and histocompatibility antigen HLA-DR3 implying a role of immunologic factors, has been reported. The disease is extremely cortisone-sensitive.

In clinical practice, TSPK is not very common but it is no rarity. In typical cases, a *confusion* with adenovirus infection is classic because of the similarity of the lesions; in atypical cases, the erroneous diagnosis tends towards herpes simplex virus infection because of the impression of branching (dendritic) figures.

At the present state of knowledge, despite all efforts to solve the riddle, TSPK remains a clinical entity with unknown origin. It is does not cause a permanent impairment of visual acuity, but its duration and unpredictable recurrences make it a source of many serious problems to the individual. It cannot be cured, but the patients can be helped by simple means. Instead of fruitless attempts to cure the keratitis with potent steroids and/or antiviral drugs and antibiotics with their well-known hazards, the symptoms can be alleviated by lubricating eye drops or, if necessary, a judicious use of low-potent steroids.

Abbreviations

Fluorescein	Fluorescein sodium
HSV	Herpes simplex virus
TSPK	Thygeson's superficial punctate keratitis
VZV	Varicella-zoster virus

The Morphology of Thygeson's Superficial Punctate Keratitis (TSPK)

5

The *smallest discernible entity* is a rounded, light-reflecting subsurface cell (about 10–15 μm in diameter). Such cells are present individually, in small groups, or aggregated in larger lesions (of about 150–400 μm in diameter, coarse lesions with the slit lamp). The nature of these cells, so clearly abnormal to the corneal epithelium, is not clear; they may represent damaged epithelial cells, invading inflammatory cells, or both.

In some of the *larger lesions* small groups of aggregated rounded/abnormal cells are discernible, in others they just seem heaped-up and/or mixed with cell debris. The lesions' shapes vary between rounded and somewhat irregular. All show rounded/abnormal cells at the edges, which thus appear rugged. The rounded/abnormal cells, whether individual or aggregated, are superficially located, but their exact location in depth cannot be estimated in two-dimensional images. The absence of changes indicating stromal involvement suggests an intraepithelial location. *Subepithelial opacities*, if developing, appeared in the present patients as a mild, transient subepithelial haze lacking abnormal cells; no informative photographs could be obtained from them.

Many rounded/abnormal cells, individual or in small groups, are present also outside the larger lesions, in *the in-between areas*. Small subsurface groups often cause surface elevations (visible as dark areas in the tear film stained with fluorescein sodium) indicating volume increase, which might be caused either by epithelial cell swelling or by the presence of additional material, such as invading inflammatory cells, or both.

Secondary phenomena manifest within the lesions as damaged grayish-whitish surface cells the light-reflecting property of which, together with that of the abnormal/rounded cells and cell debris, give the lesions a grayish-whitish appearance. *Fluorescein sodium* reveals focal surface disruptions appearing as brilliantly green dots (semi-cystic spaces) in the light-reflecting areas. The staining is always circumscript. There is no fluorescein diffusion into the surroundings or the underlying corneal stroma; adjacent surface elevations, often showing rounded/abnormal cells, appear dark in the green stained tear film. TSPK does not result in surface erosions (in the sense of loss of substance). Damaged surface cells stain red with *rose bengal* (or yellow with adherent fluorescein).

The *epithelial surface outside the lesions* is well-preserved; there is no fluorescein or rose bengal staining. In areas showing many surface elevations, the tear film stained green with fluorescein sodium appears mottled.

Epithelial cysts, some containing one or a few rounded cells, is an unspecific phenomenon occurring infrequently in typical TSPK, but many were captured in the three patients with atypical TSPK presented in Chap. 6.

Shapes and Sizes of TSPK Epithelial Lesions

Fig. 5.1 (a, b) Low-magnification photograph of TSPK epithelial lesions; in this illumination, they appear as grayish light-reflecting flecks (*arrows*)

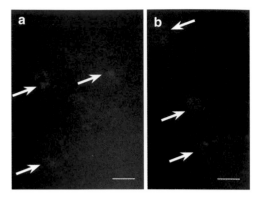

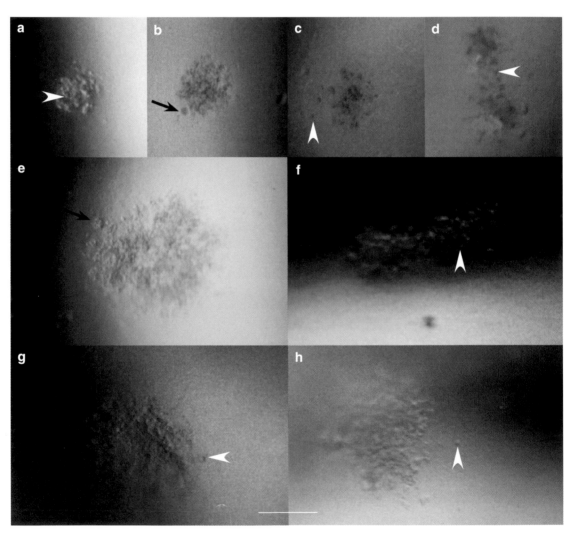

Fig. 5.2 (a–h) Various shapes and sizes of TSPK epithelial lesions. Some are rounded (a–c and e), others irregular; the club-shaped lesion in (f) seems to be a result of confluence of adjacent ones (cf. d). All lesions appear granular and have indistinct edges. Rounded/abnormal cells (*arrowheads*) are visible within and outside the lesions; some of them are aggregated in small groups (*arrows*)

Rounded/Abnormal Cells in TSPK

Fig. 5.3 (a, b) These photographs show the light-reflecting property of TSPK lesions (*arrows*). Both the rounded/abnormal cells and damaged cells/cell debris are light-reflecting

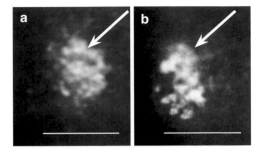

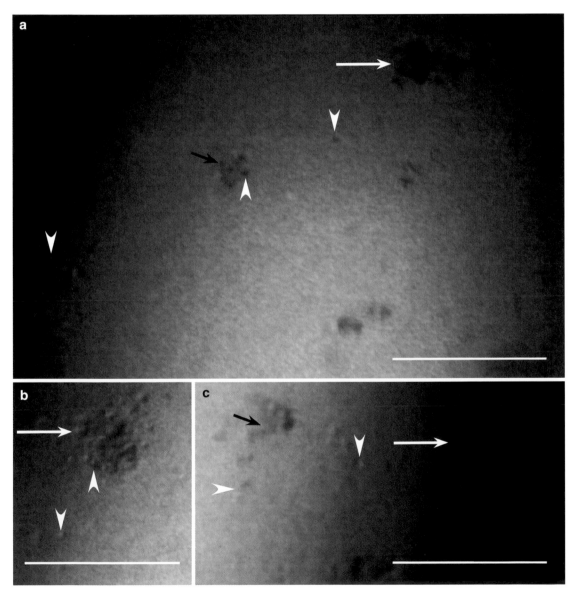

Fig. 5.4 (a–c) In this cornea with TSPK are visible many rounded/abnormal cells, individual (*arrowheads*), in small groups (*black arrows*), or aggregated in larger lesions (*white arrows*)

Fluorescein Sodium Staining of TSPK Epithelial Lesions

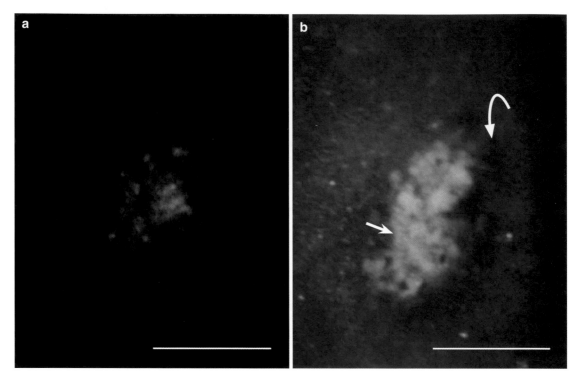

Fig. 5.5 (a) shows the light-reflecting property of a TSPK lesion. In (b) is visible circumscript green staining (partly confluent green dots; *short arrow*) indicating focal surface disruptions and penetration of fluorescein stained tear fluid into semi-cystic spaces. The periphery of the lesion is elevated (dark; *bowed arrow*); cf. also Figs. 5.6 below and 5.7, *opposite page*

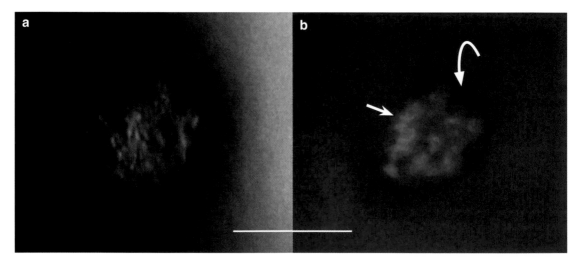

Fig. 5.6 (a, b) A TSPK lesion. (a) Without staining, it appears granular. (b) Circumscript fluorescein staining indicating fluid penetration into semi-cystic spaces (partly confluent green dots; *short arrow*); the periphery of the lesion is elevated (dark; *bowed arrow*)

Comment

For further examples of fluorescein staining see Cases; the yellow (adherent) fluorescein staining is shown in Figs. 6.9, 6.14, and 7.2

Rose Bengal Staining of TSPK Epithelial Lesions

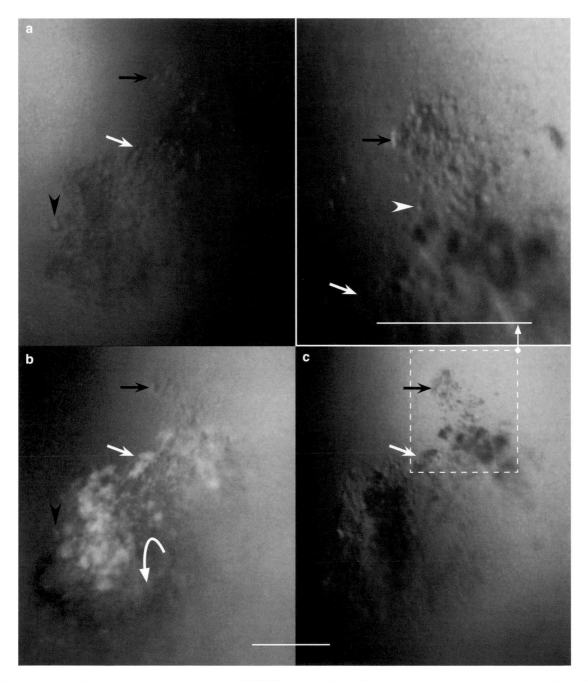

Fig. 5.7 (a–c) and *inset* show an irregularly shaped TSPK lesion that (**a**) without staining appears composed of smaller entities (*black arrow*); the *white arrow* indicates an area that is going to stain green with fluorescein (cf. **b**) and the *arrowhead* a cyst (cf. **c**). (**b**) Fluorescein shows focal surface disruptions appearing as green dots (*white arrow)* and a surface elevation (dark; *bowed arrow*); the cyst does not stain. (**c**) Red rose bengal staining demonstrates damaged surface cells/cell debris (cf. **b**). The *black arrowhead* indicates a small cyst containing a rounded cell. (The straight arrows and the black arrowheads are placed in corresponding locations.) *Inset*: the area indicated by frame in (**c**); at higher magnification rounded/abnormal cells (*arrowhead*) are visible. (The arrows are placed in the same location as in a, b)

The In-between Areas in TSPK (1)

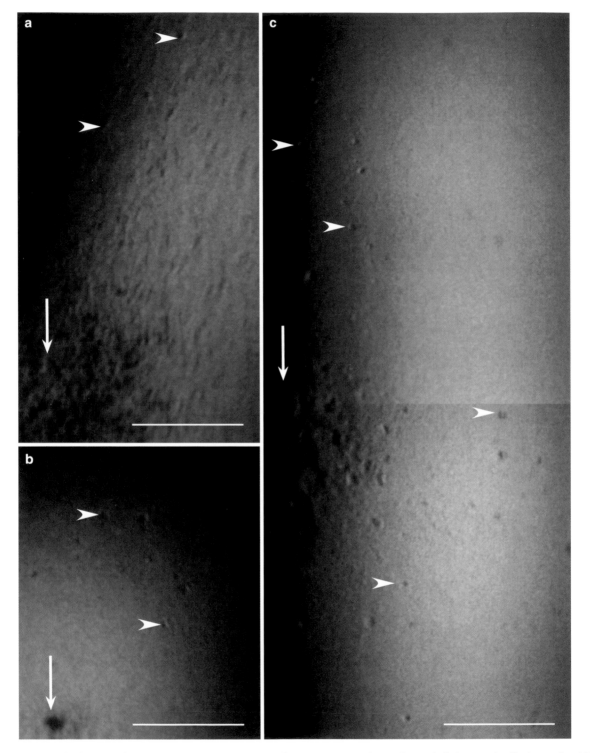

Fig. 5.8 (a–c) The areas between TSPK lesions (*arrows*) show various numbers of rounded/abnormal cells (*arrowheads*). (c is a composed photograph)

The In-between Areas in TSPK (2)

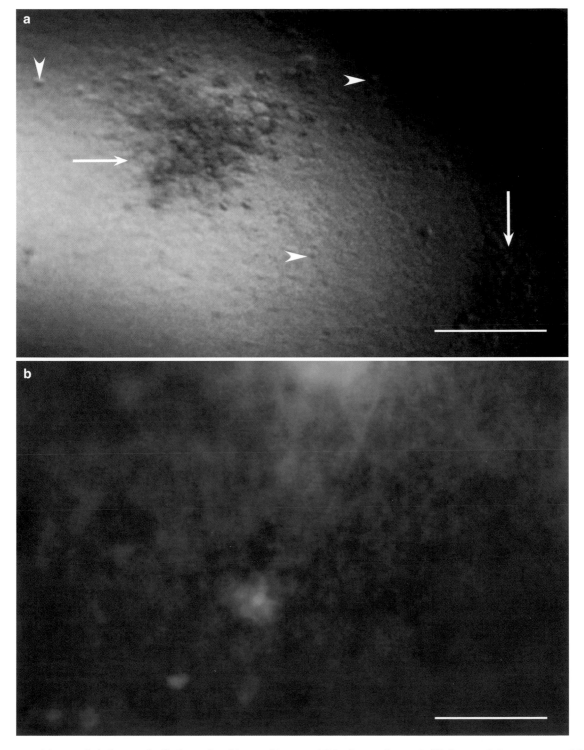

Fig. 5.9 (a) Rounded/abnormal cells (*arrowheads*) spread between TSPK lesions (*arrows*); (b) the mottled appearance of the tear film stained green with fluorescein indicates numerous slight surface elevations (*dark*). (Adapted from [1])

Typical Cases of Thygeson's Punctate Epithelial Keratitis (TSPK)

6

The four cases presented in this chapter demonstrate typical features of TSPK: the chronic, relapsing course; the common confusion with adenovirus infections; the equally common empiric use of potent topical steroids resulting in resolution of the keratitis followed by recurrence after the treatment is stopped; the presence of TSPK lesions in the absence of symptoms; and the absence of permanent damage or sight-threatening sequelae after more than two decades of the disease.

Lacking better means, the patients were treated with a weak steroid solution (prednisolone sodium phosphate 0.05%), successively tapered to almost homeopathic doses and even stopped for long periods of time. But also when symptom-free without treatment, corneal lesions were still present, with only one exception (Case 3); in this patient, 25 years after onset, the corneae appeared clear and did so also a year later. A similar event is reported in Chap. 3 (Case 3). Whether or not these patients will suffer new recurrences remains, however, open.

H.M. Tabery, *Adenovirus Epithelial Keratitis and Thygeson's Superficial Punctate Keratitis*,
DOI 10.1007/978-3-642-21634-3_6, © Springer-Verlag Berlin Heidelberg 2012

Case 1: A 24-Year History of TSPK

Case Report

A 20-year-old woman suffering from foreign body sensation, tearing, and a distressing photophobia was treated elsewhere with topical steroid, but the symptoms recurred after the treatment was stopped. At presentation, both eyes were slightly injected, and the corneal epithelium showed several grayish epithelial lesions. Topical antibiotics had no effect. All changes and symptoms disappeared rapidly with topical steroid but recurred each time after the treatment was stopped. During the following 23 years, she was treated with a weak steroid solution (prednisolone sodium phosphate 0.05%). The treatment was slowly tapered, and during the last 10 years she was using the drops only sporadically. At the last visit, 24 years after onset, she was symptom-free, but both corneae showed 10–15 TSPK lesions each.

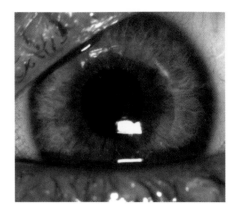

Fig. 6.1 Low-magnification photograph showing that in TSPK the eye occasionally may be injected (the patient's right eye before treatment)

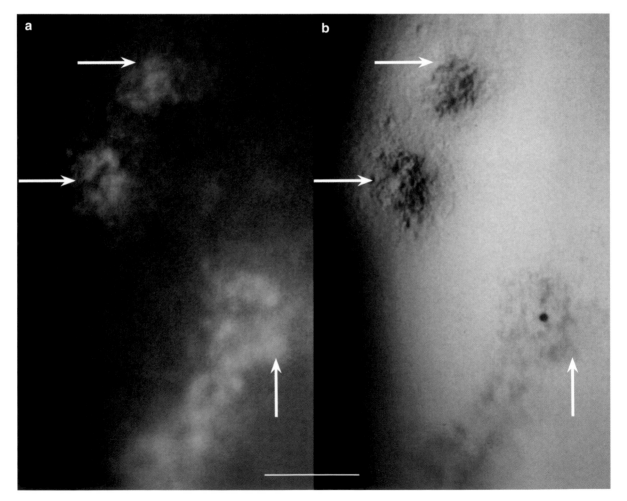

Fig. 6.2 (**a**, **b**) The cornea shows several TSPK lesions (*arrows*). In (**a**) is visible their light reflecting property and in (**b**) their granular appearance. (The arrows are placed in corresponding locations)

A 24-Year History of TSPK (Case 1, cont.)

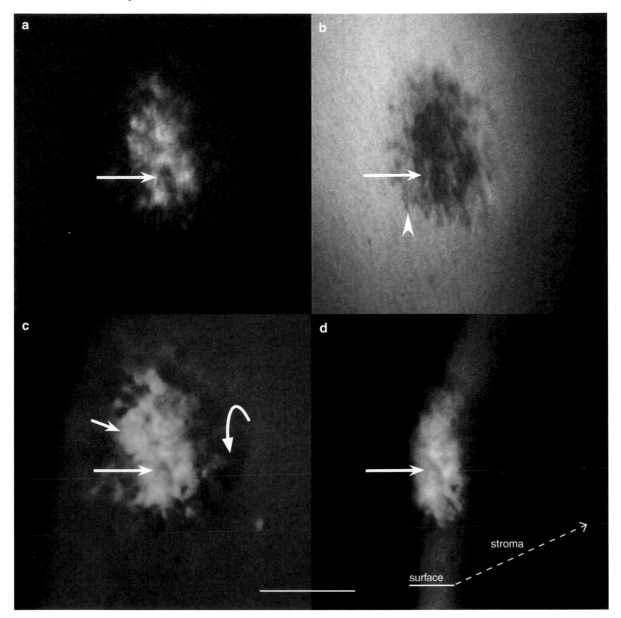

Fig. 6.3 (**a–d**) A typical TSPK lesion (*long arrows*), (**a**) light-reflecting, (**b**) appearing granular with rounded/abnormal cells visible at the edge (*arrowhead*), and (**c**) showing circumscript green fluorescein staining (*short arrow*) and surface elevations at the edge (dark; *bowed arrow*). (**d**) The superficial location of the lesion and the absence of fluorescein diffusion below the lesion is visible with a narrower light beam. (The long arrows are placed in corresponding locations in all photographs; c–d adapted from [1])

Comment

Typical of TSPK is that the eye is white but sometimes, as in this patient, the eye is injected during an exacerbation.

Case 2: A 27-Year History of TSPK with Remissions and Exacerbations

Case Report

A 36-year-old woman presented with a 6-month history of recurrent irritation, burning, and tearing in both eyes. Both corneae showed 20–30 epithelial lesions reminiscent of adenovirus infection. Eleven years later, she presented again with the same symptoms coming and going. Again, adenovirus was suspected, but the patient was referred to the Eye Clinic. Both corneae showed typical TSPK epithelial lesions. To start with, she was treated with prednisolone sodium phosphate 0.05% one or two times a day. During the following 14 years, her symptoms were minimal and she used the drops only sporadically; at each visit, the corneae showed 10–15 epithelial lesions and occasionally a few fine subepithelial opacities that faded away. When last seen, 27 years after onset, she was symptom-free without treatment despite the presence of several TSPK lesions in both corneae.

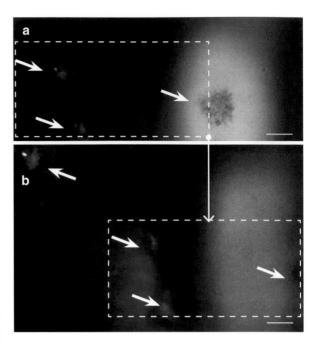

Fig. 6.4 (**a**, **b**) Survey of TSPK showing several lesions (*arrows*) (**a**) before staining and (**b**) after the application of fluorescein. The *frames* indicate the same areas

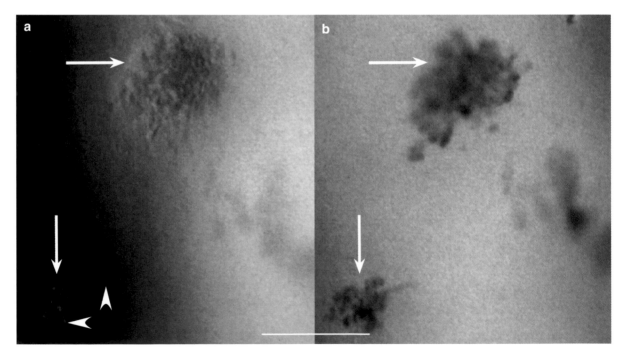

Fig. 6.5 (**a**, **b**) TSPK lesions (*arrows*). (**a**) Before staining their granular appearance and rounded/abnormal cells (*arrowheads*) within and outside the lesions are visible. (**b**) shows damaged superficial cells/cell debris staining red with rose bengal. (The arrows are placed in corresponding locations)

A 27-Year History of TSPK with Remissions and Exacerbations (Case 2, cont.)

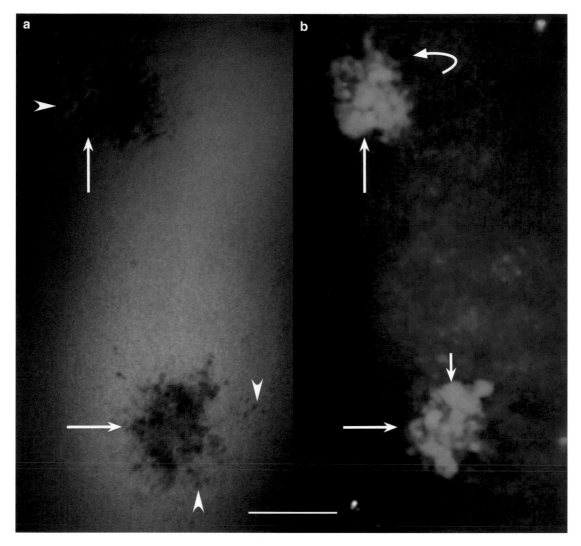

Fig. 6.6 (**a, b**) TSPK lesions (*arrows*). (**a**) shows their granular appearance and an absence of defined edges; rounded/abnormal cells (*arrowheads*) are present within the lesions and outside them. (**b**) Shows a circumscript green fluorescein staining (*short arrow*) and surface elevations (dark; *bowed arrow*). (The long straight arrows are placed in corresponding locations)

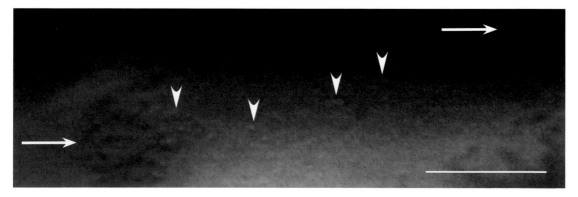

Fig. 6.7 Two TSPK lesions (*arrows*) containing rounded/abnormal cells (*arrowhead*); such cells are present also in the in-between areas (*arrowheads*)

Case 3: A Happy End (?) After 25 Years of TSPK

Case Report

A 9-year-old boy had irritation, itching, and photophobia in both eyes for a week. The eyes were white but both corneae showed many epithelial lesions that disappeared rapidly with topical cortisone. Seven years later, at the age of 16, the symptoms recurred. He was again treated with topical cortisone, for 3 months. After that, he was followed for a further 20 years. At each visit, both corneae showed several TSPK lesions, but the symptoms were minimal or none without treatment; 19 years after the onset of the second episode (26 years after disease onset), and also a year later, both corneae appeared normal.

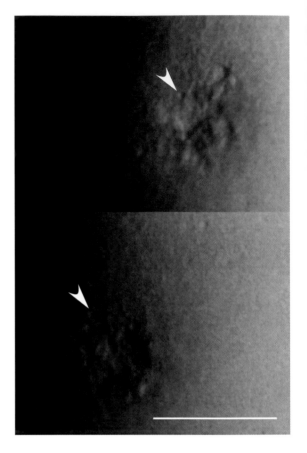

Fig. 6.8 Two TSPK lesions showing rounded/abnormal cells (*arrowheads*). (Composed photograph)

Fig. 6.9 The same lesions (*arrows*) as in Fig. 6.8. (a third one is visible to the left); they are (**a**) strongly light-reflecting, with fluorescein show (**b**) yellow (adherent) surface staining, (**c**) circumscript green staining (*short arrow*) and surface protrusions (dark; *bowed arrow*); (**d**) shows rose bengal staining of damaged surface cells/cell debris. (The long white arrows are placed in corresponding locations; c and d are composed photographs)

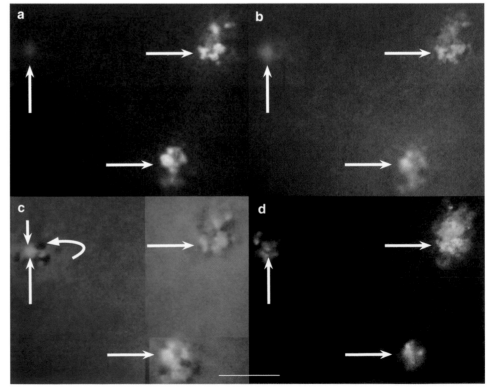

A Happy End (?) After 25 Years of TSPK (Case 3, cont.)

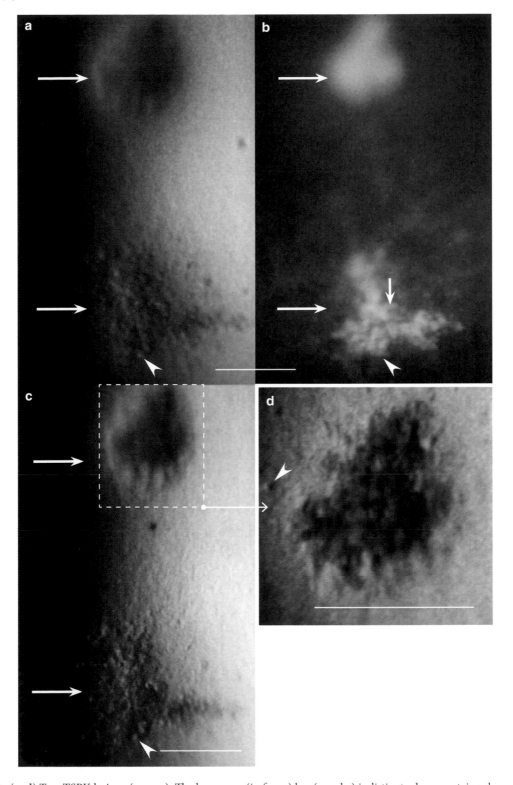

Fig. 6.10 (a–d) Two TSPK lesions (*arrows*). The lower one (in focus) has (a and c) indistinct edges, contains abnormal cells (*arrowheads*), shows (b) circumscript green fluorescein staining (*short white arrow*), and (c) red rose bengal staining of surface cells/cell debris. (d) shows the upper lesion stained with rose bengal; the *arrowhead* points to a rounded/abnormal cell. (The arrows and arrowheads in a–c are placed in corresponding locations)

Case 4: A 20-Year History of TSPK

Case Report

A 38-year-old woman with a few days' history of photophobia, tearing, and foreign body sensation in both eyes. The eyes were white but the corneae showed many epithelial lesions reminiscent of adenovirus infection. The symptoms subsided rapidly with topical steroid but returned shortly after the treatment was stopped. During the following 10 years, she was more or less continuously treated with variously potent topical steroids prescribed by various practitioners before being diagnosed with Thygeson's keratitis. During a further 10 years, she was treated with a weak steroid solution (prednisolone sodium phosphate 0.05%) and kept symptom-free with one drop every other day or twice a week. At each visit, both corneae showed a few epithelial lesions and occasionally fine subepithelial opacities, which were coming and going in various locations. The epithelial lesions were still present when last seen, 20 years after onset.

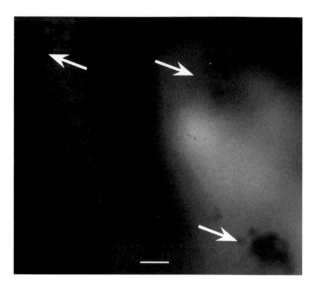

Fig. 6.11 Low-magnification photograph of TSPK lesions stained red with rose bengal (*arrows*). There is no rose bengal staining in the in-between areas

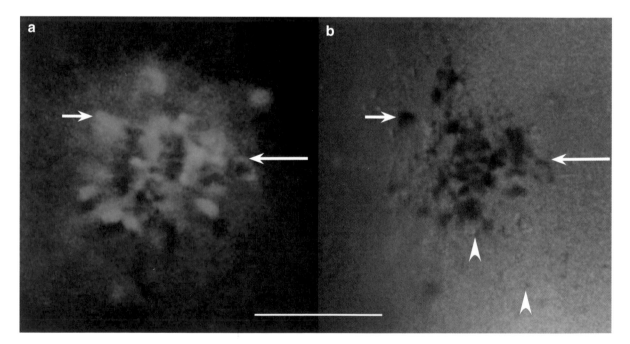

Fig. 6.12 (**a**, **b**) A TSPK lesion (*long arrows*) showing (**a**) a circumscript green fluorescein staining (*short arrow*) and (**b**) red rose bengal staining of damaged surface cells/cell debris (*short arrow*); in (**b**) are additionally visible rounded/abnormal cells (*arrowheads*). (The arrows are placed in corresponding locations)

A 20-Year History of TSPK (Case 4, cont.)

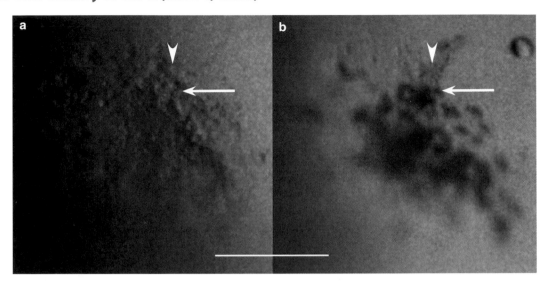

Fig. 6.13 (**a, b**) A larger TSPK lesion (*arrows*) showing rounded/abnormal cells (*arrowheads*) and (**b**) a red staining with rose bengal. (The markers are placed in corresponding locations)

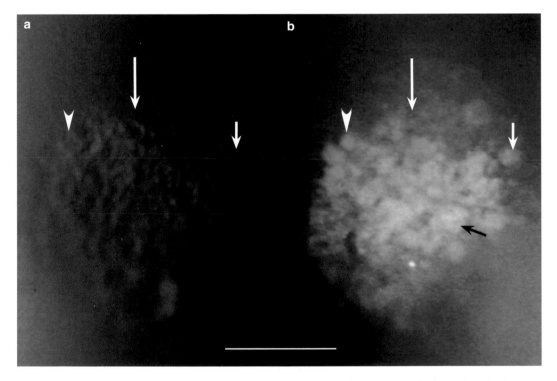

Fig. 6.14 (**a, b**) A large TSPK lesion (*long arrows*) (**a**) containing rounded/abnormal cells (*arrowhead*). The short arrow points to a spot where a green fluorescein staining is going to appear in (**b**). (**b**) shows both green (*short white arrow*) and yellow (adherent) fluorescein staining (*black arrow*). The arrowhead points to a spot in which rounded/abnormal cells are visible in (**a**). (The white markers are placed in corresponding locations; b adapted from [1])

Comment

The yellow fluorescein staining corresponds to the red of rose bengal.

Three Atypical Cases of Thygeson's Superficial Punctate Keratitis (TSPK)

7

With the slit lamp, the hallmark of TSPK are coarse granular epithelial lesions spread over the surface. The "atypical" cases are occasional patients in whom this description does not fit; yet, seen at higher magnification, the basic feature – the presence of rounded/abnormal cells within the epithelium – is the same, and so is the accompanying (unspecific) phenomenon of cysts containing one or a few rounded cells. The same history, symptoms, and the extreme cortisone sensitivity added, these patients seem to represent a variant of the same disease in which, for some reasons, the distribution pattern of the rounded/abnormal cells is more diffuse instead of the well-known distinct lesions, and the cyst are more abundant. Because of the at random confluence resulting in patterns reminding of branching (dendritic) figures, these rare cases tend to be confused with HSV rather than with adenovirus infections.

In Case 1, the pattern of epithelial changes was perhaps reminiscent of an HSV infection, but the diagnostic error could have been avoided by a more careful observation of the substructure which had no resemblance to an active HSV infection whatsoever. In Case 2, a confusion with HSV resulted in postponements of a well-needed cataract operation. Case 3 shows another variant, followed for almost 20 years. In this patient, it was notable that her granddaughter had a typical TSPK.

H.M. Tabery, *Adenovirus Epithelial Keratitis and Thygeson's Superficial Punctate Keratitis*, DOI 10.1007/978-3-642-21634-3_7, © Springer-Verlag Berlin Heidelberg 2012

Case 1: A Recurrence of an HSV Dendrite?

Case Report

A 51-year-old man was treated elsewhere with topical acyclovir for presumed HSV epithelial keratitis in the right eye. As the treatment had no effect, adenovirus was suspected and treated with topical steroid with prompt effect. A year and a half later, the symptoms recurred. Again, he was treated with acyclovir with no effect. A week later, at presentation, both corneae showed many epithelial lesions, consistent with TSPK and rapidly resolving with topical steroid. A week after the treatment was started, he had no symptoms but both corneae still showed some rounded/abnormal cells spread over the surface and a few cysts. The patient was not seen thereafter. The photographs were taken at presentation (referred to as day 1) and a week later.

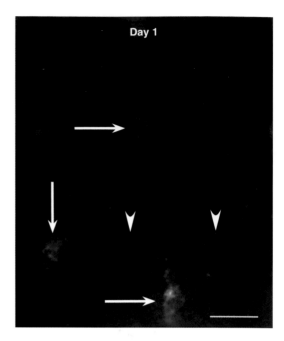

Fig. 7.1 Survey. Without staining, the cornea shows many grayish-whitish epithelial lesions (*arrows*) and light-reflecting abnormal cells (*arrowheads*) spread over the surface

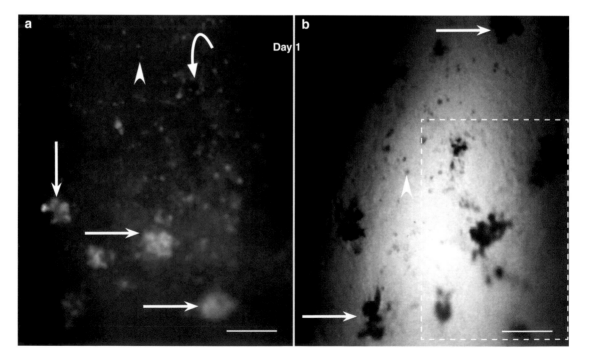

Fig. 7.2 (a) The lesions (*arrows*) stain yellow with (adherent) fluorescein and (b) red with rose bengal. In the in-between areas are visible many rounded/abnormal cells (*arrowheads*). Some areas showing rounded/abnormal cells are elevated (dark; *bowed arrow*). The area in *frame* in (b) is shown at higher magnification in Fig. 7.3 (*opposite page*). (b adapted from [1])

A Recurrence of an HSV Dendrite? (Case 1, cont.)

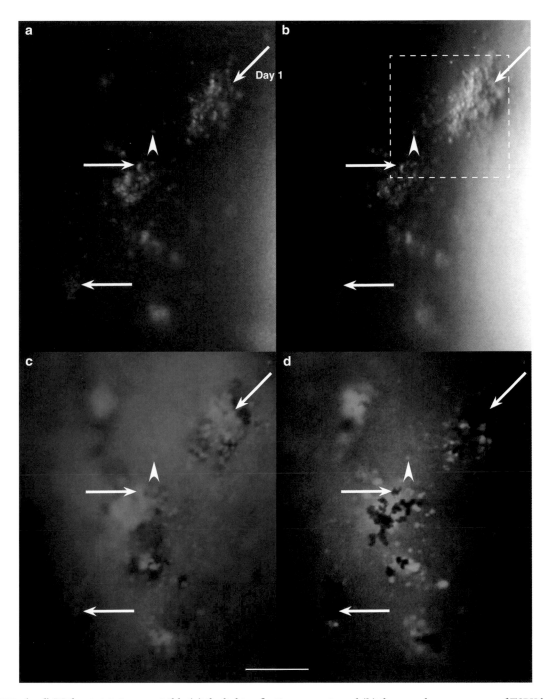

Fig. 7.3 (**a–d**) Without staining are visible (**a**) the light-reflecting property and (**b**) the granular appearance of TSPK lesions (*arrows*); (**a, b**) additionally show rounded/abnormal cells (*arrowheads*) spread in the in-between areas. (**c**) Fluorescein reveals surface elevations (dark) and brightly green dots, and (**d**) rose bengal stains damaged surface cells/cell debris. With the slit-lamp, the distribution of the lesions might give an impression of a branching figure. (The markers are placed in corresponding locations. Some other aspects of the area in *frame* in b are shown in Fig. 7.4, overleaf)

A Recurrence of an HSV Dendrite? (Case 1, cont.)

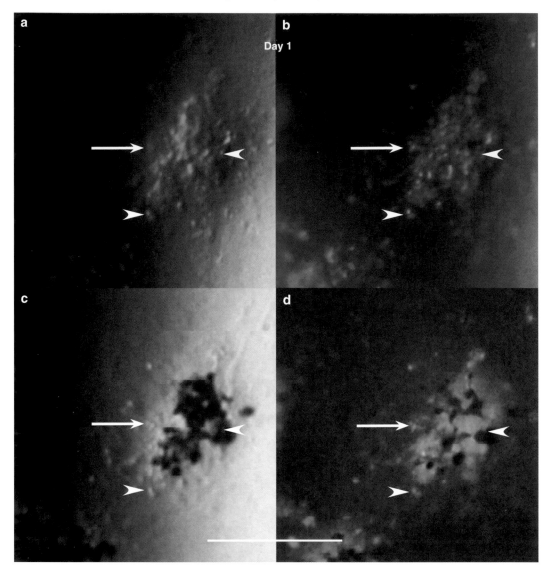

Fig. 7.4 (**a–d**) The area in frame in Fig. 7.3. Visible are: (**a–c**) many rounded/abnormal cells (*arrowheads*) giving the lesion (*arrow*) its granular appearance, (**c, d**) red rose bengal staining of damaged surface cells/cell debris, and (**d**) circumscript green fluorescein staining. The lesion has indistinct edges, and rounded/abnormal cells are present also in the surroundings. (The markers are placed in corresponding locations)

Fig. 7.5 (**a, b**) A lesion (*long arrows*) showing circumscript green fluorescein staining (the *short arrow* indicates a cystic space, cf. **b**) and a heavy rose bengal staining. Rounded/abnormal cells (*arrowheads*) are present in the surroundings. (The markers are placed in corresponding locations)

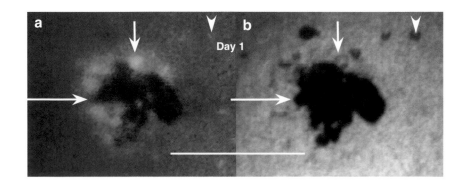

A Recurrence of an HSV Dendrite? (Case 1, cont.)

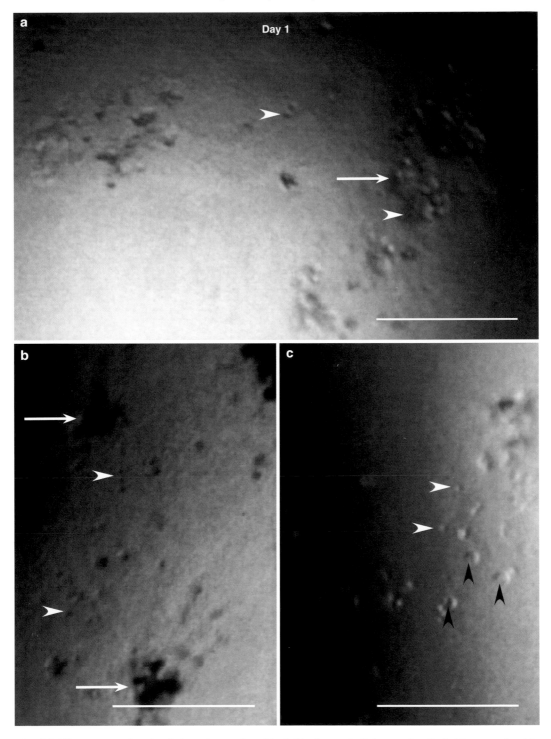

Fig. 7.6 (a–c) Different areas showing lesions (*arrows*) and individual rounded/abnormal cells (*white arrowheads*) spread over the surface. (**b** and **c**) show rose bengal staining of the lesions and the absence of red staining in the in-between areas. In (**c**) are visible rounded cysts containing rounded cells (*black arrowheads*)

A Recurrence of an HSV Dendrite? (Case 1, cont.)

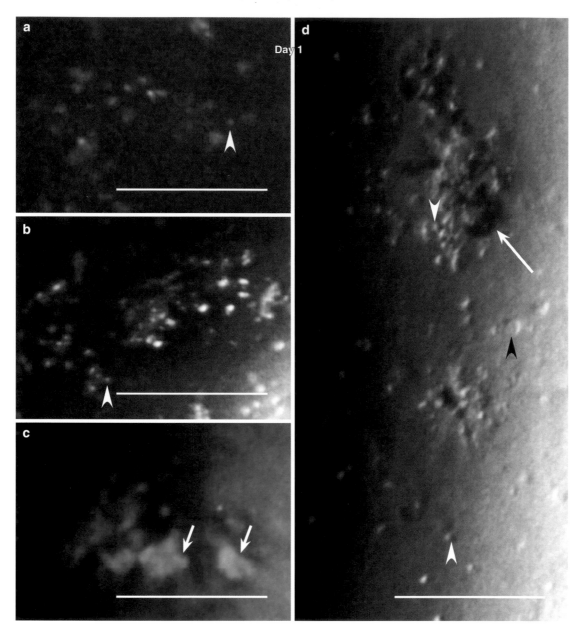

Fig. 7.7 (**a, b**) Demonstrate the light-reflecting property and the at random distribution of rounded/abnormal cells (*white arrowheads*) over the surface. In (**c**) is additionally visible a circumscript green fluorescein staining (*arrows*). (**d**) shows red rose bengal staining over an area containing heaped-up rounded/abnormal cells (*arrow*), rounded/abnormal cells (*white arrowheads*) spread over the surface, and small cysts containing rounded cells (*black arrowheads*)

A Recurrence of an HSV Dendrite? (Case 1, cont.)

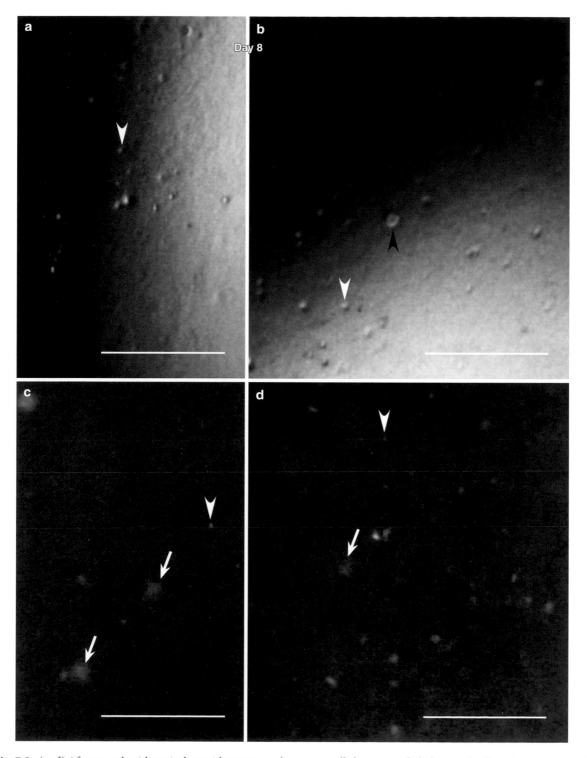

Fig. 7.8 (**a–d**) After a week with topical steroid treatment, the cornea still shows rounded/abnormal cells (*white arrowheads*) spread over the surface and green stained dots (**c**, **d**, *arrows*). In (**b**) is additionally visible a small round cyst (*black arrowhead*) containing a rounded cell

Case 2: Who Dares to Operate the Cataract?

Case Report

An 81-year-old man with a history of (presumed) recurrent herpes simplex virus (HSV) epithelial keratitis in his right eye, repeatedly treated elsewhere with topical antiviral drugs and antibiotics, was referred to Eye Clinic for cataract operation. The operation was postponed two times because of a presumably active HSV epithelial infection. At a new referral, the patient was symptom-free and the eyes white, but both corneae showed many epithelial lesions, spread over the surface and partly confluent in a pattern reminiscent of branching (dendritic) figures. He was diagnosed with (atypical) TSPK and, in the absence of symptoms, not treated with steroids. The cataract operation of the right eye was uneventful and postoperative treatment with topical steroids resulted in a disappearance of all lesions in that eye. A couple of months later, he presented because of irritation and tearing in the left eye. At that occasion, both corneae showed a few TSPK lesions. After a few days with prednisolone sodium phosphate 0.05%, the patient stopped the treatment because he was symptom-free. After that he used the drops sporadically because of recurrent symptoms. He was followed for over 2 years. The photographs taken in both corneae at various occasions show how the pattern repeats itself.

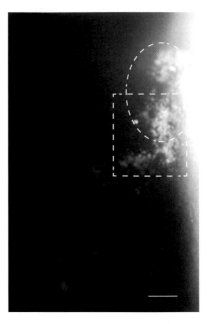

Fig. 7.9 Survey of (atypical) TSPK reminiscent of a branching figure. The area in *oval frame* is shown in Fig. 7.12 and that in *rectangular frame* in Fig. 7.13

Fig. 7.10 Also in this area, the distribution at random of rounded/abnormal cells, individual (*arrowheads*) and grouped (*arrows*), results in a pattern reminiscent of a branching (dendritic) figure

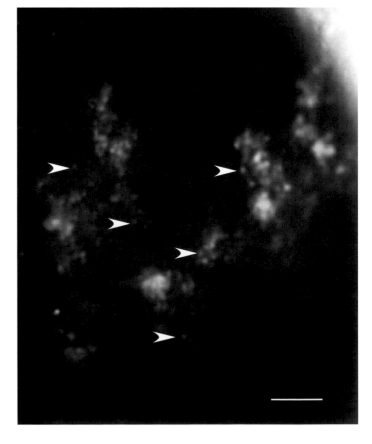

Who Dares to Operate the Cataract? (Case 2, cont.)

Fig. 7.11 Also with fluorescein, the at random distribution of the epithelial changes might be suggestive of a branching figure. Surface elevations (*bowed arrows*) appear dark in the green stained tear film; a few circumscript spaces (*straight arrows*) stain brilliantly green

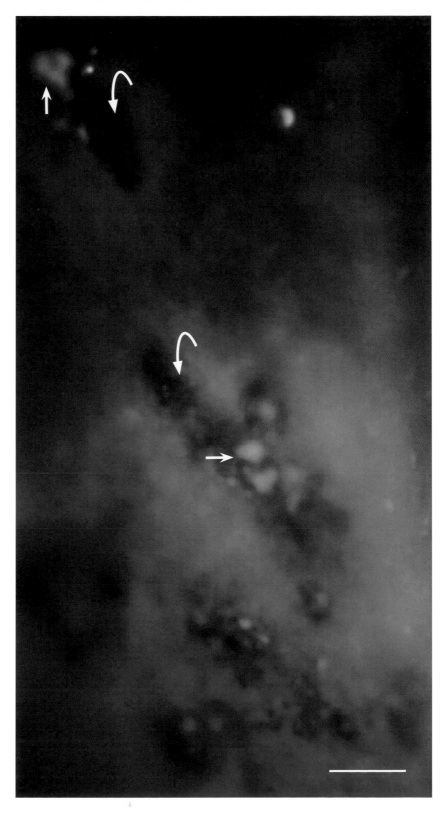

Who Dares to Operate the Cataract? (Case 2, cont.)

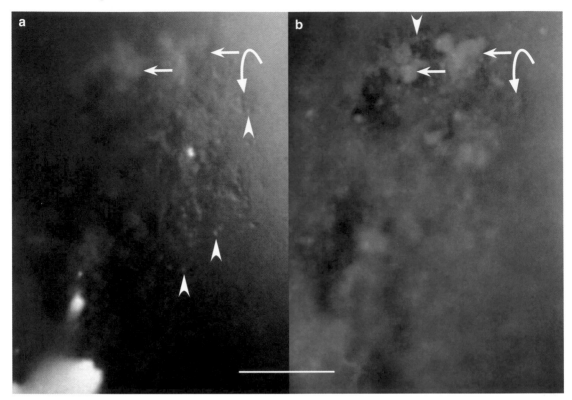

Fig. 7.12 (**a, b**) This area (indicated by oval frame in Fig. 7.9) shows surface elevations (dark; *bowed arrow*), green stained dots (*straight arrows*), and many rounded/abnormal cells (*white arrowheads*). (The arrows are placed in corresponding locations)

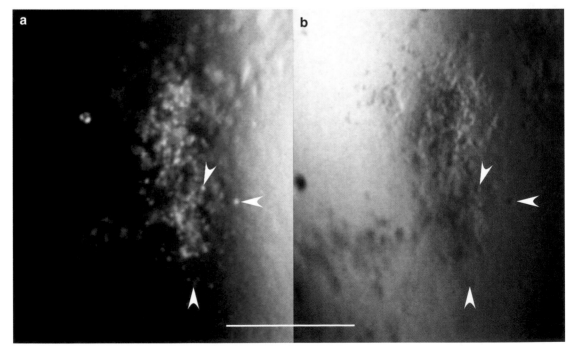

Fig. 7.13 (**a, b**) The area indicated by rectangular frame in Fig. 7.9. Visible are many rounded/abnormal cells (*arrowheads*), individual or grouped. (The arrowheads are placed in corresponding locations)

Who Dares to Operate the Cataract? (Case 2, cont.)

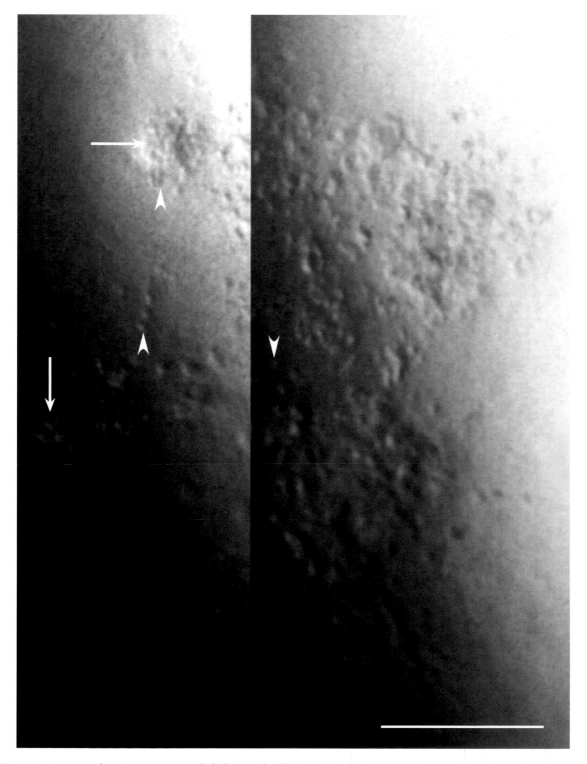

Fig. 7.14 An area showing many rounded/abnormal cells (*arrowheads*), individual, grouped, or heaped-up (*arrows*). (Composed photograph)

Who Dares to Operate the Cataract? (Case 2, cont.)

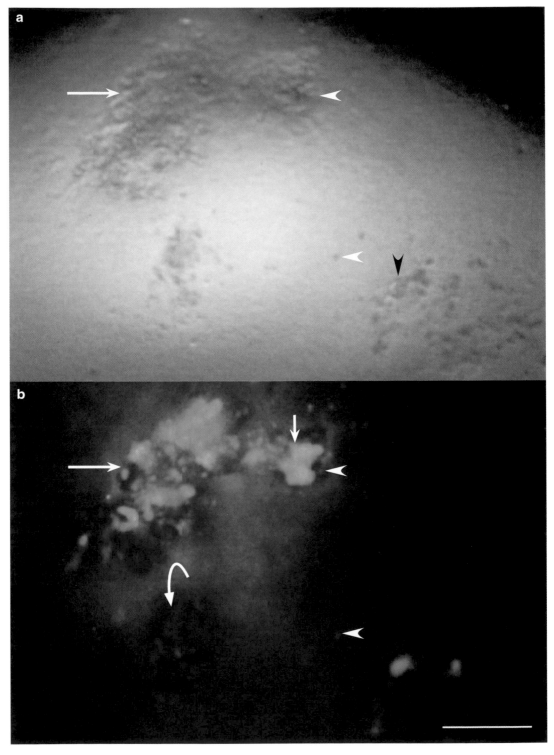

Fig. 7.15 (**a, b**) In this area, (**a**) many rounded/abnormal cells (*white arrowheads*) are in places heaped-up (*long arrows*); the *black arrowhead* indicates a cyst. (**b**) Fluorescein shows surface elevations (dark; *bowed arrow*), partly confluent brightly green dots (*short arrow*), and a green staining of the cyst (*black arrowhead*). (The arrowheads and the long arrows are placed in corresponding locations)

Who Dares to Operate the Cataract? (Case 2, cont.)

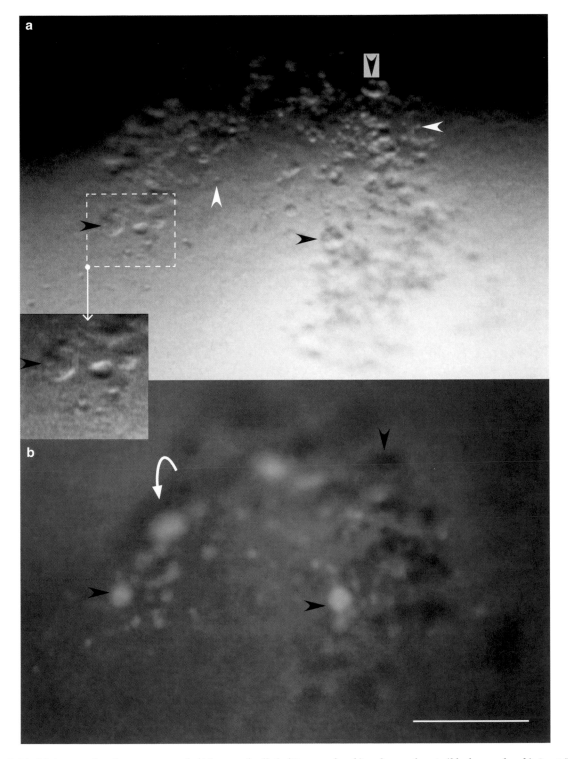

Fig. 7.16 (a) An area showing many rounded/abnormal cells (*white arrowheads*) and several cysts (*black arrowheads*). *Inset*: The cyst within the area in *frame* contains rounded cells. (b) Some cysts (*black arrowheads*) stain green with fluorescein, others do not stain; the *bowed arrow* indicates a surface elevation (*dark*). (The black arrowheads are placed in corresponding locations)

Who Dares to Operate the Cataract? (Case 2, cont.)

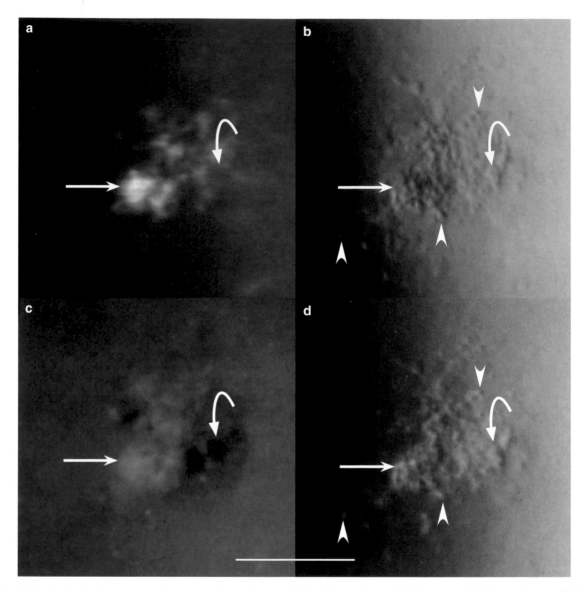

Fig. 7.17 (**a**–**d**) At this occasion, the cornea showed a typical TSPK lesion (*arrow*). The lesion is (**a**) light-reflecting, (**b**) has indistinct edges and contains rounded/abnormal cells (*arrowheads*). (**c**) shows surface elevations (dark; *bowed arrowhead*) in the green stained tear film, and (**d**) patches of yellow surface staining (*straight arrow*) with fluorescein. In (**b** and **d**) are additionally visible rounded/abnormal cells (*arrowheads*) in the surroundings. (The markers are placed in corresponding locations)

Who Dares to Operate the Cataract? (Case 2, cont.)

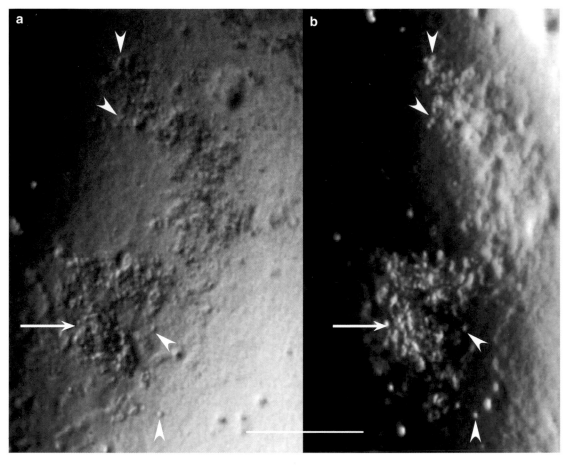

Fig. 7.18 (a, b) The same area captured in different illumination modes. The at random arrangement of rounded/abnormal cells, individual (*arrowheads*), grouped (*black arrow*), or heaped-up (*white arrow*) gives an impression of a continuous figure. (The markers are placed in corresponding locations; adapted from [1])

Fig. 7.19 An area showing rounded/abnormal cells (*white arrowhead*), individual or heaped-up (*arrows*), and round cysts (*black arrowheads*)

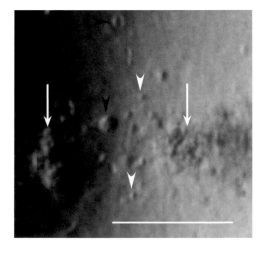

Case 3: A Peculiar Epithelial Keratitis

Case report

A 57-year-old woman with irritation in the left eye, which started a month before in conjunction with a febrile illness, presented because of blurred vision in her right eye for about a week. The eyes were white. Both corneae showed fine dust-like light-reflecting opacities, spread in dendritiform patterns and apparently located in the deeper epithelial layers. Her symptoms were mild and treated only with lubricating eye drops. Within 7 weeks, her visual acuity returned to normal, the right cornea still showed some cysts and dots, and the left one appeared normal. Virus isolation test was negative for HSV and adenovirus and immunofluorescence test from conjunctival scraping negative for adenovirus.

The photographs of the right cornea were taken on day 1 (at presentation), day 8, and day 15, and after 4 and 7 weeks.

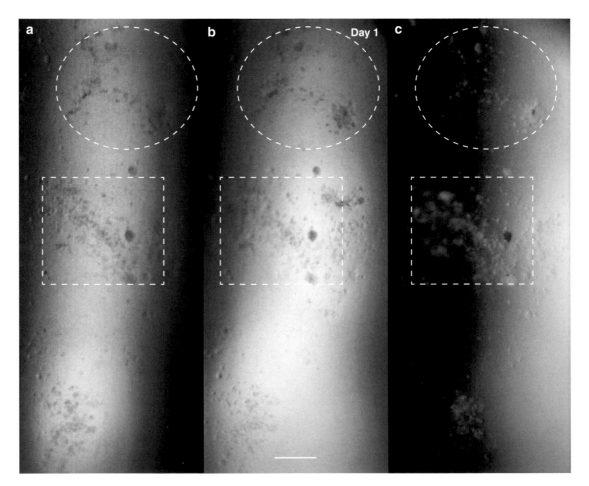

Fig. 7.20   (a–c) Survey of corneal epithelial changes captured on day 1 (at presentation), (a) without staining, (b, c) after application of fluorescein, and (c) with addition of rose bengal dye. The patterns are reminiscent of branching figures. The area in *oval frame* is shown at higher magnification in Fig. 7.21 (*opposite page*) and that in *rectangular frame* in Fig. 7.22 (*overleaf*)

A Peculiar Epithelial Keratitis (Case 3, cont.)

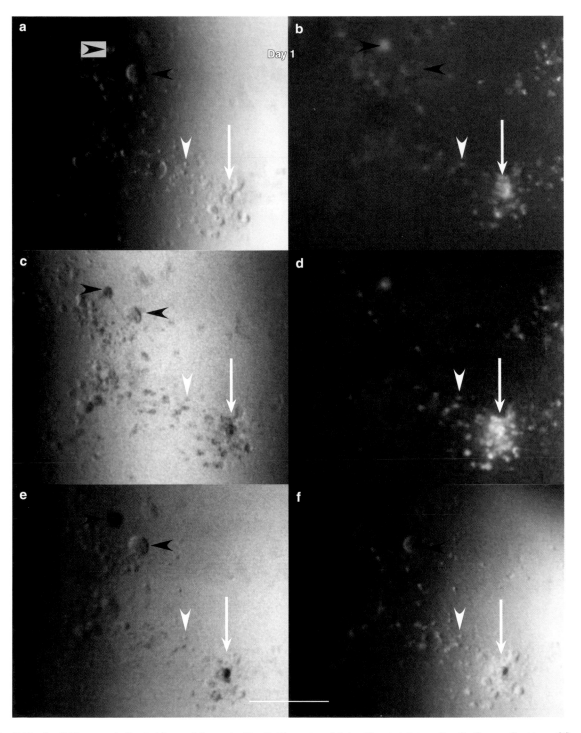

Fig. 7.21 (**a–f**) The area indicated by oval frame in Fig. 7. 20, captured (**a**) without staining, (**b–d**) after application of fluorescein, and (**e–f**) after addition of rose bengal, shows many rounded/abnormal cells (*white arrowheads*). Of the two small cysts (*black arrowheads*), the left stains both with fluorescein (**b–d**) and rose bengal (**e–f**); the right one does not stain. The *arrow* indicates an area suggestive of a TSPK lesion. (The markers are placed in corresponding locations)

A Peculiar Epithelial Keratitis (Case 3, cont.)

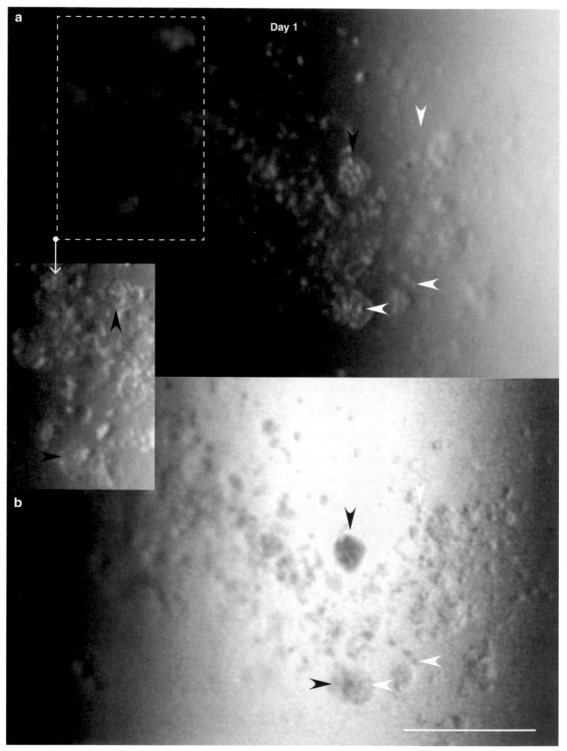

Fig. 7.22 (a–d) (This and opposite page). Also this area, indicated by rectangular frame in Fig. 7.20, shows many rounded/abnormal cells (*white arrowheads*), the arrangement of which implies a branching figure, and several cysts (*black arrowheads*) containing rounded cells. Of the cysts staining with fluorescein (**b**, inset in **a**, **b**, and **c**) the majority stains also with rose bengal (**d**, inset in **c**, **d**). There is no fluorescein diffusion into the epithelium and no rose bengal surface staining except for the cysts. (The markers are placed in corresponding locations)

A Peculiar Epithelial Keratitis (Case 3, cont.)

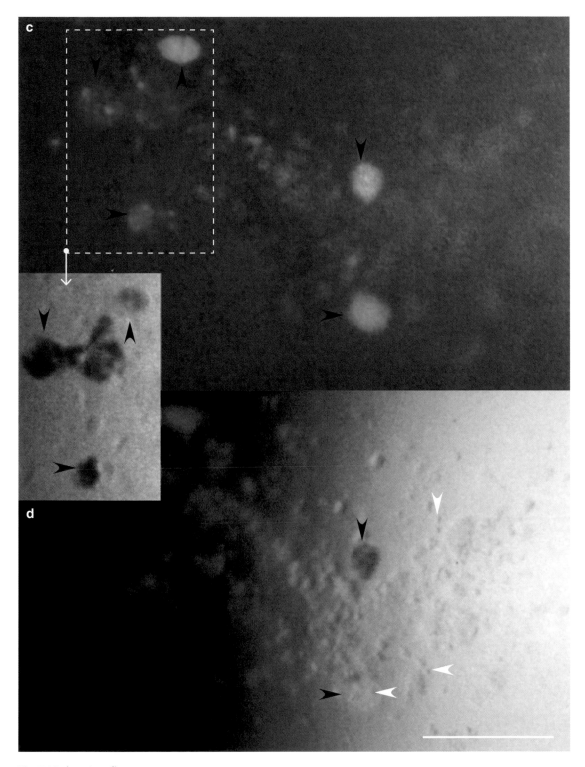

Fig. 7.22 (continued)

A Peculiar Epithelial Keratitis (Case 3, cont.)

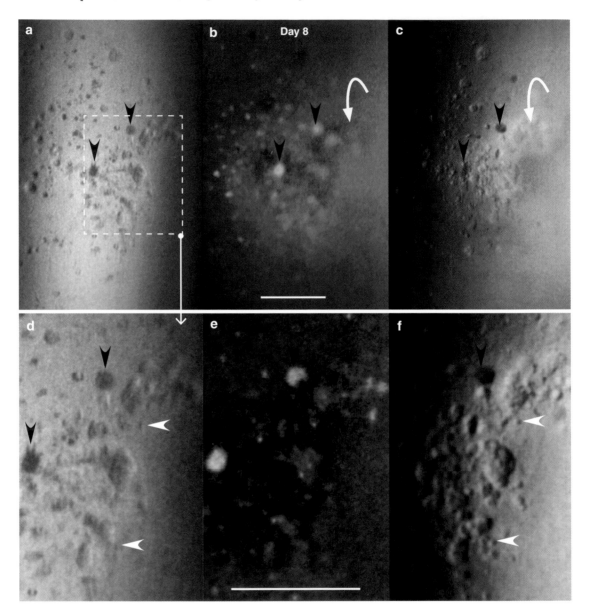

Fig. 7.23 (**a–f**) Day 8. The same area captured after staining with fluorescein (**a, b; d, e**) and rose bengal (**c, e,** and **f**). (**a–c**) Survey. The *black arrowheads* indicate cysts staining with fluorescein and rose bengal. The area in frame is elevated (dark in the green stained and pale in the red stained tear film; *bowed arrowheads*). (**d–f**) The area indicated by frame in (**a**) at higher magnification; visible are many rounded/abnormal cells (*white arrowheads*) and several cysts. (**e**) There is no fluorescein staining except for the cysts. (The markers are placed in corresponding locations)

Fig. 7.25 (**a, b**) (*Opposite page*). Day 15. Two photographs capturing the same area in slightly different illuminations. In both are visible rounded/abnormal cells (*white arrowheads*) and several cysts (*black arrowheads*) containing rounded cells. (The arrowheads are placed in corresponding locations)

A Peculiar Epithelial Keratitis (Case 3, cont.)

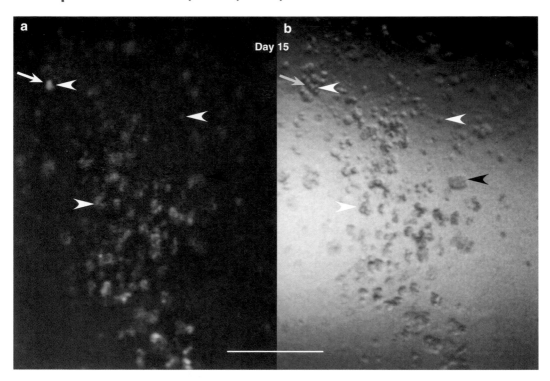

Fig. 7.24 (**a, b**) On day 15, the epithelium still shows many rounded/abnormal cells (*white arrowheads*), individual or in small groups, epithelial cysts (*black arrowhead*), and a few dots stained green with fluorescein (*arrow*). (The markers are placed in corresponding locations)

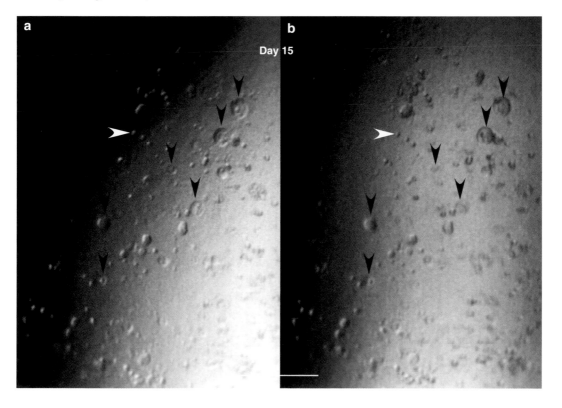

A Peculiar Epithelial Keratitis (Case 3, cont.)

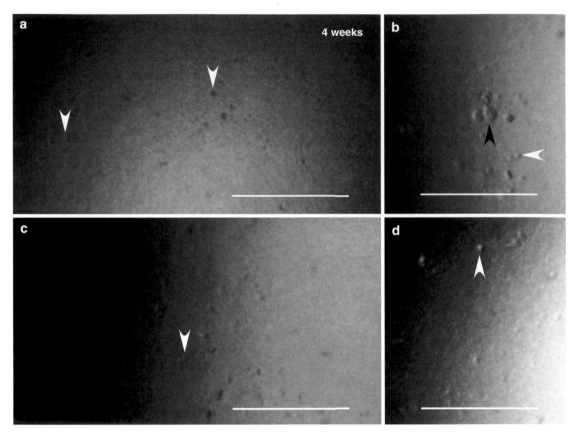

Fig. 7.26 (**a–d**) Four weeks after presentation, the epithelium shows rounded/abnormal cells (*white arrowheads*) spread over the surface. In (**b**) is additionally visible a group of small cysts (*black arrowhead*)

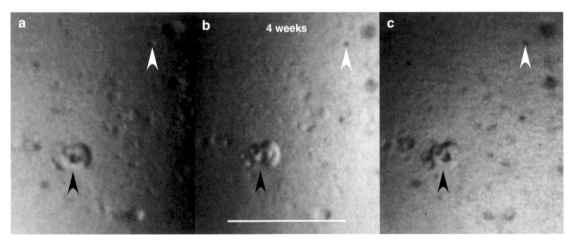

Fig. 7.27 (**a–c**) Three photographs capturing the same area show a cyst (*black arrowheads*) containing rounded cells and individual rounded/abnormal cells (*white arrowheads*). (The arrowheads are placed in corresponding locations)

A Peculiar Epithelial Keratitis (Case 3, cont.)

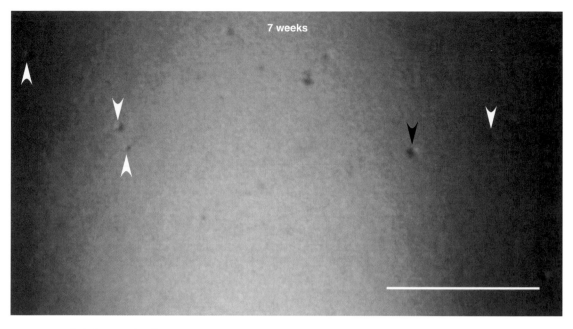

Fig. 7.28 Rounded/abnormal cells (*arrowheads*) spread over the surface are still present 7 weeks after presentation. The rounded structure indicated by the *black arrowhead* might represent an incipient cyst

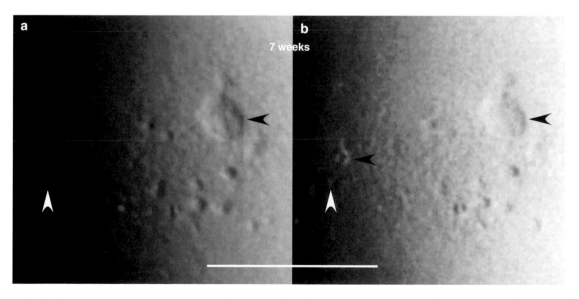

Fig. 7.29 (a, b) A small area showing rounded/abnormal cells (*white arrowheads*) and cysts (*black arrowheads*) 7 weeks after presentation. (The markers are placed in corresponding locations)

A Peculiar Epithelial Keratitis (Case 3, cont.)

About *16 months later,* the symptoms recurred in the *left eye.* The eye was white, and the cornea showed the same type of opacities as at the previous occasion. The patient was diagnosed with atypical TSPK. The symptoms resolved spontaneously within 5 weeks. The right eye remained uninvolved.

The photographs of the left cornea were taken at various occasions.

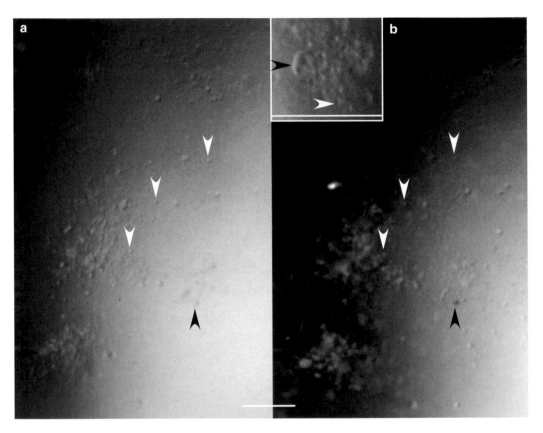

Fig. 7.30 (a, b and inset) During this second attack, the corneal epithelium shows, again, many rounded/abnormal cells (*white arrowheads*), individual and grouped, and rounded cysts (*black arrowheads*) staining with fluorescein (a, b) and some also with rose bengal (b). (The arrowheads are placed in corresponding locations)

Fig. 7.31 (a, b) This area (*arrow*) containing rounded/abnormal cells (*white arrowhead*) and a cyst (*black arrowhead*) reminds of a TSPK lesion. Rounded/abnormal cells are present also outside the lesion (*upper white arrowhead*). (The markers are placed in corresponding locations)

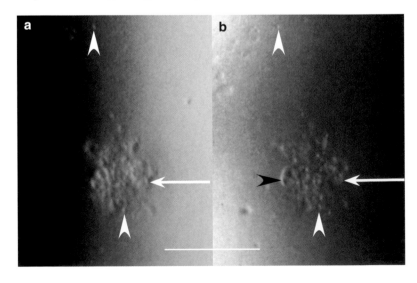

A Peculiar Epithelial Keratitis (Case 3, cont.)

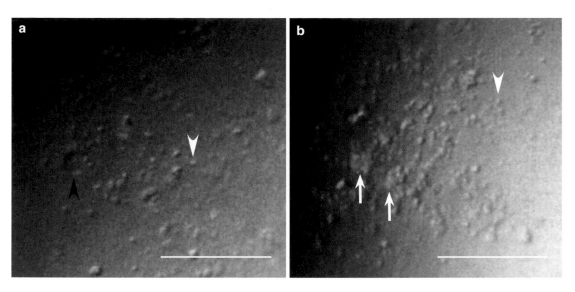

Fig. 7.32 (**a**, **b**) Two different areas both showing many rounded/abnormal cells (*white arrowheads*). In (**a**) is additionally visible a cyst (*black arrowhead*) and in (**b**) a minimal fluorescein staining (*arrows*)

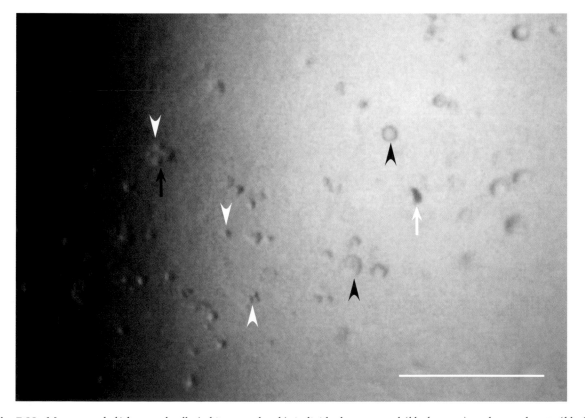

Fig. 7.33 Many rounded/abnormal cells (*white arrowheads*), individual or grouped (*black arrow*), and several cysts (*black arrowheads*) spread over the surface. There is a minimal rose bengal staining (*white arrow*)

A Peculiar Epithelial Keratitis (Case 3, cont.)

After a *further 10 months* (now 2.5 years after onset), the symptoms recurred in *both eyes*, starting as one small group of epithelial opacities in the right eye and two in the left one. The opacities spread over both corneae and disappeared within 1 month.

The photographs of both corneae were taken at presentation and of the right one also 10 days later.

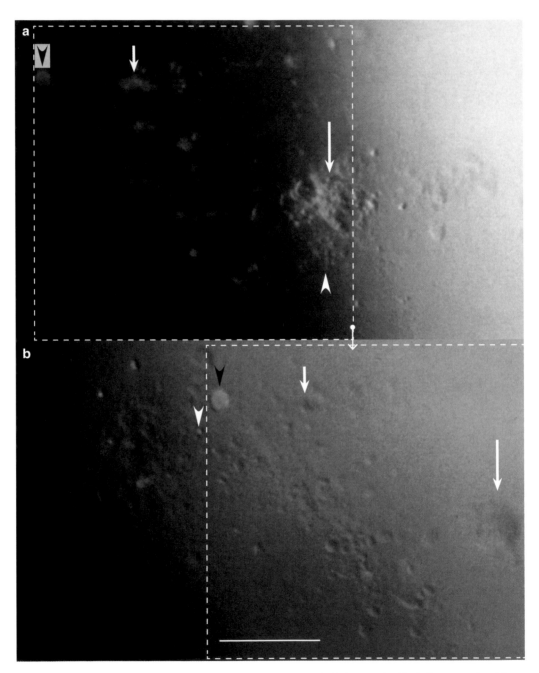

Fig. 7.34 (**a, b**) The epithelium of the right cornea shows many rounded/abnormal cells (*white arrowheads*), in one area heaped-up (*long white arrow*). A cyst (*black arrowhead*) stains green with fluorescein; the *short white arrow* points to one of several spots staining yellow with (adherent) fluorescein. Rose bengal was not used. (The *frame* indicates the same area shown in a and b; the arrows and the black arrowheads are placed in corresponding locations; a adapted from [1])

A Peculiar Epithelial Keratitis (Case 3, cont.)

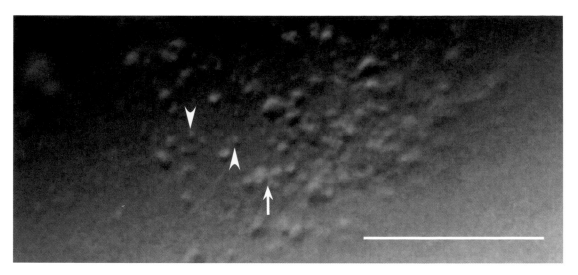

Fig. 7.35 This area of the right cornea shows many rounded/abnormal cells (*white arrowheads*) and a minimal fluorescein staining (*arrow*)

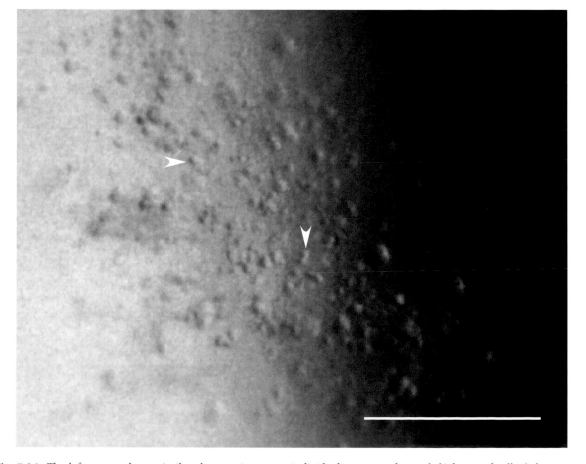

Fig. 7.36 The left cornea shows similar changes, i.e., many individual or grouped rounded/abnormal cells (*white arrowheads*); the *black arrowheads* indicate epithelial cysts

A Peculiar Epithelial Keratitis (Case 3, cont.)

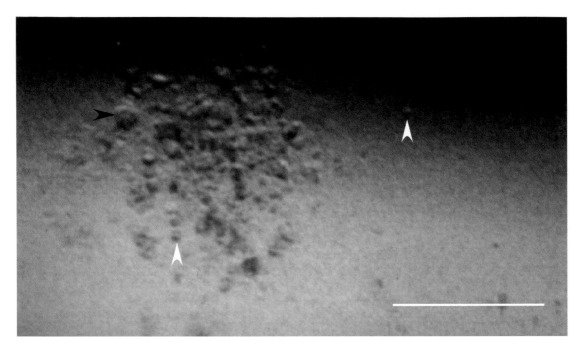

Fig. 7.37   Ten days later, the right cornea shows rounded/abnormal cells (*white arrowheads*), partly concentrated in a rounded area and partly present outside it. The black *arrowhead* points to a cyst

Addendum 1

A fourth attack occurred *one year later* (over 3.5 years after onset) in the left eye; the symptoms subsided spontaneously within 2 months, but the corneal changes did not completely disappear. Four months later, the right eye suffered a new attack, and shortly thereafter the opacities spread again over the left cornea. The keratitis was waxing and waning but never disappeared completely in either eye, for 9 months. After that, the more affected right eye was treated with prednisolone sodium phosphate 0.05%, and the keratitis resolved rapidly. The keratitis persisted in the left eye but the patient had no symptoms. Later on, because of blurred vision, she started to use the drops once daily also in the left eye, and the keratitis resolved. A month later, while she was using the drops every other day, the keratitis recurred in the right eye with very little symptoms. She did well on low-dose steroid. Two

years had elapsed after the onset of this period before both corneae were clear and the treatment stopped. Thereafter the patient was seen every 6 months, had no symptoms, and both corneae remained clear.

Over 5.5 years later (now about 11.5 years after onset), the symptoms recurred in the left eye and rapidly resolved with prednisolone sodium phosphate 0.05%, once daily. During the following 8 years, she did well without treatment and there was no recurrence.

The patient was found to have dry eye (break-up time 1–2 s, Schirmer 1 test 2 mm of wetting in 5 min, the test repeated at several occasions during remissions) but no dry eye related corneal epithelial changes. Both corneae additionally showed endothelial changes (cornea guttata). She had no associated general illness.

When the patient had the third attack of eye symptoms, she asked me to see her granddaughter. To my surprise, the girl had a typical TSPK. The history and findings are reported here (*opposite page*).

Addendum 2. Typical TSPK in a Relative

Case Report

The patient, a filial granddaughter of a patient with atypical TSPK (referred to as Case 3 in this chapter), was a 9-year-old girl with symptoms of recurrent eye irritation, tearing, and photophobia, all starting at the age of 6. As far as known, her symptoms had started a couple of months before her grandmother's. A medical record, dated a year before presentation, described bilateral keratitis in white eyes resolving with topical cortisone. At presentation, both corneae showed several typical TSPK lesions; the same picture was observed two and four years later. Since her symptoms were mild and of short duration, no cortisone was used. At the age of 15, when last seen, both corneae were clear. Since then, as reported by her grandmother, the girl had no symptoms.

The patient's mother reported that the girl was healthy except for a history of alopecia at the age of 7, a problem that remained unexplained and resolved spontaneously. She had varicella about 3 years after the onset of ocular symptoms.

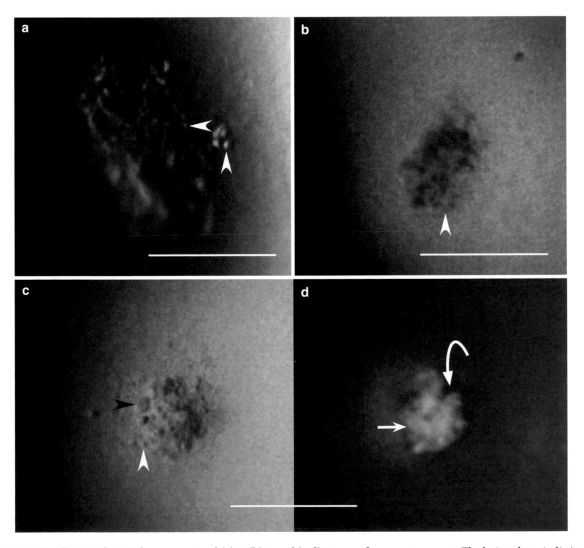

Fig. 7.38 (a–d) Typical TSPK lesions captured (a) 3, (b) 5, and (c-d) 7 years after symptom onset. The lesions have indistinct edges and show heaped-up rounded/abnormal cells (*white arrowheads*). In (a) and (c) are additionally visible small cysts (*black arrowheads*) and in (d) a circumscript green fluorescein staining (*short arrow*) and elevated edges (dark; *bowed arrow*) (c, d adapted from [1])

Final Remark

In the interpretation of in vivo ocular surface changes, whether in clinical setting or at higher magnification, a *comparison* between disturbances caused by various agents is indispensable. Finding common and diverging features is helpful not only in differential diagnostics but also in understanding of the mechanisms behind them. In adenovirus infections, it seems natural to compare the morphology with that due to infections with the two other major viruses causing human epithelial keratitis, *HSV and VZV*. A comparison, however, is only partly possible. The reason is that in adenovirus infections the *route of virus access* to the epithelium is external, corresponding to that of primary HSV and VZV infections; the problem is that these primary infections are rare in an adult, and thus the experience with a primary HSV infection captured by the same method is limited to one case [6] and that with VZV is, unfortunately, none. (In retrospective, referring to the only case of primary HSV infection, the initial confusion with adenovirus could have been avoided by paying attention to the early appearance and the composition of epithelial foci, neither of them compatible with adenovirus.) Still, keeping in mind that in recurrent HSV and VZV infections the virus reaches the corneal epithelium via the corneal nerves which results in a focal involvement, some comparison can be made.

The three infections *differ* in that the *in vivo virus CPE* is easily discernible in both HSV and VZV but, strangely enough, not so in adenovirus infections. It may be that in the latter, during the acute stage, a sure identification of the virus CPE comparable to that in vitro is hampered by a diffuse epithelial involvement per se also compatible with unspecific oedematous changes.

A feature all three have *in common* is the presence of *rounded/abnormal cells* which, as already mentioned (Chap. 1) may represent incipient cell swelling, cells with damaged membranes for other reasons, or invading inflammatory cells; by the present method, these alternatives are indistinguishable from each other. In *HSV and VZV* keratitides, such cells are discernible in areas of a previous epithelial involvement after the disappearance of the overlying epithelial disturbance relatable to the virus CPE, and thus it seems reasonable to assume that they represent invading inflammatory ones. Because preceded by overlying changes disturbing their detection, the point of time when they start to appear cannot be determined. In *adenovirus* infections, the interpretation calls for prudence because in the absence of a preceding epithelial focus of infection there is nothing to relate their locations to, their visibility is undisturbed, and their appearance coincides with the infectious stage of the disease; it is possible but remains to be proven that in adenovirus epithelial keratitis invading inflammatory cells are a very early occurrence.

Connected with this question is another feature common to all the three infections – *focal corneal epithelial involvement*. In *HSV and VZV*, it is the first sign of the disease; it is related to the route of infection via the corneal nerves; it clearly shows the virus CPE; and it either disappears with treatment (HSV) or shows typical spontaneous changes (VZV). Nothing like that occurs in *adenovirus epithelial infiltrates*: they start to appear several days after symptom onset, form against a background of a diffuse epithelial involvement, lack features indicating the virus CPE, have a uniform appearance in which no signs suggestive of ongoing virus infection can be discerned, and persist after the acute stage had subsided. These diverging features

H.M. Tabery, *Adenovirus Epithelial Keratitis and Thygeson's Superficial Punctate Keratitis*,
DOI 10.1007/978-3-642-21634-3, © Springer-Verlag Berlin Heidelberg 2012

imply that HSV and VZV focal lesions and adenovirus epithelial infiltrates are of different origin. In adenovirus infiltrates, long-term observations of their dynamics in conjunction with comparison with TSPK shed some light on the possible mechanisms behind their development (below).

In all the three infections, as a sequela, *subepithelial opacities* may develop which later on, without knowledge on the cause, could be attributed to any of them.

The morphology of *TSPK lesions* highlights why the *confusion with adenovirus* infections is so common. If two comparable photographs – one showing an adenovirus epithelial infiltrate and the other a typical TSPK lesion – were put in front of you, I wonder if you could tell which is which. I do not think I could. As far as can be discerned, both contain many rounded/abnormal cells, concentrated in a small area and overlain by damaged superficial epithelial cells.

This *similarity* implies the same type of reaction. In *TSPK*, the situation is simple: The keratitis appears as if from nowhere and either persists indefinitely or disappears spontaneously only to recur later on or, hopefully, never. This behaviour, and the sensitivity to cortisone, implies an immunologic disorder. (In a way, the course of TSPK reminds of some cases of idiopathic anterior uveitis).

In *adenovirus* infections, on the other hand, the sequence of events can be followed, from the initial stage during which the presence of living virus on the ocular surface can be proven to the sequelae of the infection. This late stage shows subepithelial infiltrates the disappearance of which with topical steroids, and their reappearance after the treatment is stopped, is a well-known phenomenon that, similarly to TSPK, implies an involvement of immunologic factors. When exactly during the course of the disease they start to operate seems unknown, but tracing back the morphology hints at an early event. The development of epithelial infiltrates in the presence of living virus on the ocular surface does not necessarily indicate that they are the result of a direct virus impact on epithelial cells because there is a distinct possibility of an overlap of two events of which one (relatable to the action of infectious virus) is manifest while the other (relatable to immunologic responses) is starting to show. The sequence of events shows that, with time, the first ceases while the other continues. Indeed, this would explain why the morphology of adenovirus epithelial infiltrates is so dissimilar to focal lesions caused by living viruses (HSV and VZV) but so similar to TSPK. In both diseases, the morphology of the lesions is well compatible with heaping-up of extraneous material (rounded/abnormal cells) mixed with damaged epithelial cells proper. In TSPK, the presence of inflammatory cells has been shown in *histological preparations*.

In both adenovirus infections and TSPK, the lesions in question are only the tip of the iceberg. With the slit lamp, the *in-between areas* seem inconspicuous, but they also show rounded/abnormal cells yet without any other associated epithelial disturbance. Probably, these cells are eliminated by transportation towards the surface from which they are shed, and the epithelial architecture is visibly disturbed only in places in which, for some reasons, they are concentrated. That the distribution of the rounded/abnormal cells varies and occasionally shifts towards more diffuse patterns show the "atypical" TSPK cases. (Actually, "atypical TSPK" is a misnomer because doubtfully "punctate," but unless some other important feature distinguishing it from typical TSPK is found, there is hardly a need for inventing a new terminology.)

Hence, it seems that corneal epithelial infiltrates in adenovirus infections and "coarse" TSPK epithelial lesions are the result of the same reactive process which, however, may be an unspecific one, i.e., provoked by different agents. In adenovirus infections, the virus antigen is the primary suspect; in TSPK, despite all efforts to identify it, the agent remains unknown. It may be that it is not to be found among the known ones, or it has never been there when tested.

Index

H.M. Tabery, *Adenovirus Epithelial Keratitis and Thygeson's Superficial Punctate Keratitis*,
DOI 10.1007/978-3-642-21634-3, © Springer-Verlag Berlin Heidelberg 2012

Printing and Binding: Stürtz GmbH, Würzburg